ANIMALS, DISEASE AND HUMAN SOCIETY

In recent years, the issue of animal disease has seldom been out of the headlines. The emergence of BSE and the threat of food-borne infections such as *E. coli* and salmonella have focused public attention on the impact of animal disease on human society. However, the problem of animal disease is far from new. *Animals, Disease and Human Society* explores the history and nature of our dependency on other animals and the implications of this for human and animal health.

Writing from a historical and sociological perspective, Joanna Swabe's work discusses such issues as:

- animal domestication;
- the consequences of the human exploitation of other animals, including links between human and animal disease;
- the rise of a veterinary regime, designed to protect humans and animals alike;
- the implications of intensive farming practices, pet-keeping and recent biotechnological developments.

This account spans a period of some ten thousand years, and raises important questions about the increasing intensification of animal use for both animal and human health. All those interested in human–animal relationships or in public health issues will find *Animals, Disease and Human Society* a thought-provoking and rewarding work.

Joanna Swabe is a Postdoctoral Researcher affiliated to the Amsterdam School for Social Science Research, Amsterdam, The Netherlands.

ROUTLEDGE STUDIES IN SCIENCE, TECHNOLOGY AND SOCIETY

1 SCIENCE AND THE MEDIA
Alternative routes in scientific communication
Massimiano Bucchi

2 ANIMALS, DISEASE AND HUMAN SOCIETY
Human–animal relations and the rise of veterinary medicine
Joanna Swabe

ANIMALS, DISEASE AND HUMAN SOCIETY

Human–animal relations and the rise of veterinary medicine

Joanna Swabe

ROUTLEDGE

London and New York

First published 1999
by Routledge
11 New Fetter Lane, London EC4P 4EE

Simultaneously published in the USA and Canada
by Routledge
29 West 35th Street, New York, NY 10001

Typeset in Garamond by Routledge
Printed and bound in Great Britain by
TJ International Ltd, Padstow, Cornwall

British Library Cataloguing in Publication Data
A catalogue record for this book is available from the British Library

Library of Congress Cataloguing in Publication Data
Animals, disease and human society: human-animal relations and the rise of veterinary medicine / Joanna Swabe.
Includes bibliographical references and index.
1. Veterinary medicine – History. 2. Domestic animals – Social aspects – History. 3. Human – animal relations – History. 4. Zoonoses – History. I. Title
SF 615.5935 1998
98 – 25860
636.089`09 – dc21 CIP AC

ISBN 0–415–18193–3

CONTENTS

Acknowledgements vi

1 Introduction 1

2 Domestication, dependency and disease 19

3 Animals, disease and human social life: from ancient times to the early modern period 50

4 The unfolding veterinary regime 85

5 The intensification of livestock production and the veterinary regime during the twentieth century 118

6 Pandering to pets: pet-keeping and the emergence of small-animal practice 156

7 Epilogue 192

Appendix 206
Notes 212
Bibliography 217
Index 233

ACKNOWLEDGEMENTS

Every book has its own history. This one originally began life as a doctoral dissertation at the Amsterdam School for Social Science Research, University of Amsterdam under the title of *The Burden of Beasts*. While researching and writing this volume I benefited greatly from the moral support and practical advice provided by all my friends and colleagues at the Amsterdam School. I am especially grateful to Joop Goudsblom and Bart van Heerikhuizen for their enthusiastic supervision and support of my work. Throughout the past few years, I have profited immensely from their wisdom, guidance and encouragement. I would also like to acknowledge Anneke van Otterloo, Fred Spier and Nico Wilterdink of the University of Amsterdam for their insightful comments and critique of the final manuscript; and Peter Koolmees and Jan van Logtestijn of the Faculty of Veterinary Medicine at the University of Utrecht for going over the veterinary and veterinary historical content of my work with a fine-tooth comb. Likewise, I am grateful to Juliet Clutton-Brock, Liliane Bodson and James Serpell for their invaluable comments on Chapters 2, 3 and 6 respectively; and also to the various veterinarians who afforded me access to their busy practices in the earliest stages of my research.

Naturally, I would also like to thank my family and close friends for their support. My parents, Eve and Tony Swabe, have always encouraged my academic endeavours and undoubtedly will be proud of this volume, as will the rest of my kith and kin; most particularly my grandparents, Sid and Cissie Gasson, to whom it is dedicated. My special thanks also go out to Hella Steins and Mieke van Stigt who have helped me get through the writing process more or less intact; and to Ian Macdonald for being my long-suffering partner in crime. Finally, this book about human–animal relations would not be complete without mention of the non-human creatures that share my life. I have learned much about the nature of the relationship between people and pets from living under the same roof as three fiendish felines. In fact, strange as it may seem, it is perhaps to Apie, an elderly black-and-white tom, that I owe the greatest debt of gratitude. Were it not for the inordinate amount of time and money that I have spent on him at the vet's, I might never have hit upon the idea of taking the veterinary profession as my subject of study at all.

1

INTRODUCTION

On animals we depend

In modern industrial society, where everyday existence often seems completely divorced from the natural world, it is all too easy for we humans to ignore the extent of our dependency on other animals. For the denizens of the great urban sprawls that typify the modern age, encounters with animals tend to be quite minimal. In towns and cities, the only animals that prevail are those that lurk around our homes and gardens as pets, those wild birds that inhabit the polluted skies and the vermin that creep stealthily through the sewers. Occasionally, the odd police horse may impinge upon this urban landscape, or a city farm might bring the sights and sounds of the countryside within arm's reach. However, the closest that the average urban dweller will usually get to a chicken, cow, pig or sheep in everyday life is when they pluck a vacuum-packed cut of meat from the refrigerated shelves of the local supermarket for the evening meal. Even then, it is likely that they will be scarcely aware of – or will even question – the origins of their food. The animal form will have been carefully concealed in colourful and hermetically-sealed packaging, often with all traces of blood, vessels and fats removed. Alternatively, it may have been enshrouded in crispy crumbs or bathed in delectable sauces or marinades, disguising the meat still further. In today's world, it is extremely easy to dissociate the product that is consumed from the living, breathing and feeling creature from whence it came (Fiddes 1991).

We are in fact dependent on animals to provide most of the protein that we consume. Meat, dairy produce and eggs constitute a significant part of the modern western diet. At times these animal products are eaten to excess; sometimes there is a reluctance to consume them at all. In recent years, for example, health concerns have increasingly led to an apparent decline in the consumption of red meat and an increase in poultry and fish eating. Furthermore, an increasing sensitivity to animal welfare and environmental issues has led more and more people to reject the consumption of meat and fish altogether. Vegetarianism is currently enjoying increasing popularity, although only a small proportion of those who stop eating meat will also cease to consume animal-derived protein altogether. Even when animal flesh has been excluded, dairy produce and eggs will often continue to play an important role in the vegetarian diet.[1] However, our dependence on animals to provide a large proportion of our food does not simply stop at the provision of meat, milk and eggs.

The modern western diet is a highly complex one that is greatly reliant upon manufactured foods. A supermarket today is like an Aladdin's cave where one can find everything that one's heart and stomach desires. From gourmet microwave meals to mouth-watering cakes, biscuits and pastries, literally hundreds of ready-made food products line the shelves to entice the consumer. But what goes into these products? How are they made? Take, for example, confectionery; a packet of, let us say, wine gums may seem completely innocuous until one takes the trouble to read the label. High on the list of ingredients one is likely to find reference to a substance called 'gelatine'. These tasty sweets may seem somewhat less appetising when one realises that gelatine is in fact a thickener that is obtained by boiling the skins, tendons, ligaments and bones of slaughtered animals (Ockerman and Hansen 1988: 132–57). At first glance, confectionery bears very little relationship to cattle, but the link is very often there. In reality, much of the manufactured food that we today ingest is not always of such obvious animal origin; so much so that even the most committed of vegetarians can end up consuming by-products of the slaughterhouse unwittingly. Unless one has an encyclopaedic knowledge of ingredients and food additives, falling foul of slaughterhouse by-products is easy. Moreover, reading labels is also far from infallible; a substance, such as glycerine, can derive either from the abattoir, or from vegetable sources.

Our dependency on animals as the providers of food thus goes far beyond simply the production of meat, milk and eggs; what remains of the animal after it has been used in life and its quality edible parts removed after death is essential to the production of manufactured foods. Slaughtered animals are generally exploited to the full and the substances obtained from dead animals are a valuable source of income for farmers and abattoir owners (see Appendix, Tables 2, 3 and 4). After slaughter, precious little of the animal is wasted: the fats, gelatine, glycerine, rennet and collagen commonly found in food are all generally derived from slaughtered animals. Glycerine, for instance, is used as a humectant (moistener) and solvent for other food additives. Rennet, an enzyme with coagulant properties used in the manufacture of cheese, is obtained from the stomachs of slaughtered calves (Ockerman and Hansen 1988: 198). Collagen too derives from the connective tissue from meat, and is found in food and also, more commonly, cosmetics. Even the E numbers that are found almost ubiquitously in manufactured food may derive from animals. Food additives, such as emulsifiers, stabilisers, thickeners and glazing agents, can often be of animal origin. In addition to these slaughterhouse by-products, one may find other animal ingredients such as lactose and lecithin that are derived from milk and eggs respectively. Even those vegetarians who enjoy a tipple might be unpleasantly surprised to discover that their favourite beverage contains rather more than just alcohol. Beer conditioned in casks, for instance, requires fining to clear the yeast which is suspended in the liquid during the brewing process. Isinglass, a substance derived from the bladders of sturgeon, is commonly used to perform this task. Similarly, wine production also involves fining: isinglass, gelatine, egg albumen, casein, chitin (from the shells of crabs and lobsters) and, in the past, even ox blood have been commonly used for this purpose (Bowler 1990: 110–11).[2]

Further to food, we are also dependent on animals for their natural fibres and hides. Textiles made from wool provide us with warmth and floor coverings, animal hair and bristles are used to make brushes and hide to make shoes, clothes, furniture, sports equipment and even cleaning cloths. Parchment and vellum are also made from animal skin. Animal fur is not only used to make coats and hats, but can also be found on children's toys. Duck and goose down is used to fill pillows, duvets and sleeping bags, and feathers used to decorate hats or make quills for calligraphy. Animal bones are used to make high-quality china goods. Further to this, animal fats from the slaughterhouse, such as tallow, can be used to produce cheap candles and soap. Other abattoir by-produce is commonly found in cosmetics. Moisturising creams, for instance, often contain collagen or the animal proteins reticulin and elastin; hair conditioners are made using keratin, an animal protein obtained from wool or the slaughterhouse. Stearates are also used as emollients in creams and lotions, as well as in lipsticks, shampoos and as emulsifiers for perfumes. Additionally, lanolin, a substance obtained from the grease found on sheep wool, is often found in cosmetics. It may surprise many people to learn that although their cosmetics may not necessarily have been tested on animals, they nonetheless contain ingredients that often derive from the slaughterhouse. Likewise, photography is entirely dependent upon gelatine for processing. Unlike many other ingredients, there is no alternative to this substance if one wishes to make photographic prints (Ockerman and Hansen 1988: 152). Even the medicines that we ingest or inject are often of animal origin: e.g. insulin, amino acids, oestrogen, progesterone, testosterone, steroids and, less frequently, vitamin B12 and calcium (Ockerman and Hansen 1988: 176–200). Garden and agricultural fertilisers may also contain dried blood and bone-meal, in addition to animal manure (Kotula 1991). Finally, animal remains are commonly rendered down and used to make feed for agricultural animals. The wisdom of feeding herbivores on the remains of other creatures, however, has recently come into question in the light of the emergence of bovine spongiform encephalopathy (BSE), the so-called 'mad cow disease' (Fisher 1997; Lacey 1994).

In the modern world, we are also highly dependent on animals to test the safety and reliability of many of the products that we use in our everyday lives. Animals are commonly employed in laboratory settings to gauge the potential toxicity of ordinary household products such as shampoos, detergents, toothpaste, washing powder, glues, pesticides, cosmetics and toiletries, in addition to testing for the kind of eye and skin irritation such products may possibly cause. Even the cigarettes to which a substantial proportion of the western population are addicted have also been tested on animals during the course of their development and manufacture. Animals have also been used by the military to assess and improve the effectiveness and impact of modern weaponry. The physical effects of poisonous gases, radiation and bullets have, for example, been appraised through the use of animals. Likewise, animals have also made useful tools for psychological research, providing behavioural data from which, for example, human mental processes have been imputed (Singer 1990: 25–94). Furthermore, animal testing is more or less standard in the pharmaceutical industry. Before medicines are deemed safe for human use, they are required under governmental regulations to undergo stringent tests. In the earlier stages of development, such tests will often involve gauging the drug's effect and potency in animals. Even the vaccines and drugs employed for veterinary use will generally have undergone extensive tests for quality control on laboratory and target animals in order to ensure their safety for use on other animals (van der Kamp 1994). While alternatives have been developed that, in some circumstances, obviate the need for experimentation on live animals – and, in recent years, the numbers and kinds of animals used for experimentation have been significantly reduced – animal use within the biomedical and life sciences remains commonplace. Irrespective of changes in attitudes and scientific practices, the scientific and medical research community still have a vested interest in perpetuating animal experimentation given the employment opportunities it offers for both researchers and technicians.

Aside from their roles as the providers of edible and useful ingredients and as the tools of science, animals in our society are also commonly used for entertainment and recreational purposes. Zoological gardens and wildlife parks, for instance, provide us with the opportunity to observe exotic and often dangerous wild animals. Likewise, we also turn to television, which has taken the animal kingdom as one of its favourite subjects to enlighten and entertain. We visit circuses to watch animals perform death-defying feats and attend gymkhanas, horse races and dog tracks to see – and sometimes even bet on – the skill and speed with which animals can move at human command. Equine mounts are also saddled up for pure recreation. Cantering on horseback through the countryside or parks is a pastime that many enjoy; some even using these animals to indulge themselves in yet another 'sporting pleasure' involving other creatures, namely the hunting and killing of foxes and deer. Horseriding may also be used to assist the therapy of disabled and handicapped people, particularly children; such 'hippotherapy' has been found to have significant emotional and physical benefits (CSS report 1988: 36–7). We even enjoy riding on the backs of trussed-up donkeys when we visit the seaside. Animals are also kept recreationally as a hobby; cat and dog fanciers attend shows to eagerly parade and win prizes for the specimens that they have painstakingly bred and groomed, while those keeping or collecting more unusual pets such as reptiles, insects and ornamental fish often belong to specialist clubs and societies that service their animal interests. Caged birds and aquaria are also kept purely for ornamental purposes, as decoration for homes, restaurants, offices and other public places (CSS report 1988: 3–5). As we shall see later in this volume, animals are also widely kept by people as pets for a wide variety of reasons, the most significant of which being the pure companionship that they can offer. On a more perverse note, animals may sometimes serve a rather dubious recreational function as the subjects of pornography and sexual delight (Dekkers 1992).

Finally, we are reliant on animals to perform highly specific tasks within our society. Dogs, in particular, have been found to have a multitude of working uses throughout the ages. Sheepdogs have for centuries been trained to herd and protect flocks of sheep. Likewise, large and powerful breeds, such as Alsatians, Dobermans and Rottweilers, have been frequently employed to guard and protect private property. Today, the police and military services also commonly use Alsatians in their routine work to intimidate and apprehend suspects. Furthermore, police, military and customs authorities employ smaller and specially trained 'sniffer' dogs in order to search for illegal drugs and explosives. The canine sense of smell and the species' great tractability have also made them useful helpers in the rescue of trapped and injured people after accidents and disasters. The ability to track and retrieve prey is also an age-old character trait that has to this day made the dog a favourite hunting partner for humans. Throughout the past few decades, canines have increasingly been used to help humans as guide dogs for the blind, hearing dogs for the deaf and as service dogs for the disabled. Horses are today also employed as working animals, generally by the police and military. Sometimes their use is purely ceremonial, but with their size and brute force they are often utilised for crowd control and for surveillance purposes.

This catalogue of animal usage is by no means exhaustive. There are many more ways in which we depend on animals in our everyday lives, not all of them as practical as those uses listed above. We should not, for example, underestimate the important role that animals have often played in cultural thought and practice. As various anthropologists have been keen to point out, animals possess a great symbolic power and the way in which they have been represented in various cultures, including our own, has influenced both the manner in which we view human identity and think about other species (e.g. Douglas 1966; Lévi-Strauss 1966; Ingold 1988; Willis 1990). Animals are, it seems, not only good to eat, but also 'good to think' (Harris 1985a; Tambiah 1969). The power of animal symbolism and representations can clearly be found today in the animal imagery that pervades today's society through the mass media, advertising and film (Baker 1993). We are also dependent on animals to enrich our language: animals provide powerful metaphors with which we can describe others, in addition to being the source of a whole host of extremely effective insults on which we can depend to cause our fellow humans emotional injury (Leach 1964; Fiddes 1991).

About *Animals, Disease and Human Society*

This book is primarily about our species' great dependency on other animals. It is about the way in which animals have been manipulated and used to service human needs, desires and requirements throughout human history. More importantly, this book is about the serious repercussions that humankind has had to face as a consequence of its ever-increasing and intensifying exploitation of animals. When I speak of animal exploitation, I do not intend it in any kind of derogatory or moralistic sense: this book is most definitely *not* about animal rights or human wrongs. Although the moral status of animals within human society is a very important issue indeed, it has not been the specific focus of my work. More to the point, I feel that it is a subject that has already been dealt with more than sufficiently in the existing literature on the human–animal relationship. The philosophical, political and ethical aspects of the rights of animals have, for example, been extensively and intelligently discussed by authors such as Peter Singer (1990), Mary Midgley (1983) and Tom Regan (1984); while the more sociological angle on the subject of animal rights has already been covered by Keith Tester (1991). My aim, as a sociologist, is to provide as dispassionate a view as possible of our relationship with other animals, rather than to become embroiled in political and moral debate. In this respect I have used the expression 'animal exploitation' throughout this volume in its very strictest sense, i.e. that we derive benefit from utilising animals to our own ends. Indeed, it is my view that humans tend to regard animals as a natural resource; they provide us with a reliable, continual and self-renewing supply of the protein, hide, natural fibres, manure and muscle power, etc., on which we depend (Swabe 1996). It is my contention that the exploitation of animals has become part of – what Pierre Bourdieu (1984) has described as – our *habitus*; in other words, it is a principle that the vast majority leave unquestioned in their everyday lives.

The apparently tacit assumption that humans have the prerogative to exploit other creatures to their own ends has in fact found a great deal of concrete support throughout the history of European society, most particularly within the teachings of the Judaeo-Christian tradition. According to the biblical narrative of Genesis 1:

26–8 and Genesis 9: 2–3, humankind's right to have dominion over and subdue other living creatures was a God-given one. Human ascendancy over the natural world was, thus, taken to be part and parcel of the divine plan. Under the influence of such theological rationalisations, animals were simply understood by people to be there, and specially designed by the creator, to serve specific human purposes. In this regard, Keith Thomas cites one early eighteenth-century physician who went so far as to argue that God even made 'horse's excrement smell sweet, because he knew that men would often be in its vicinity' (Thomas 1983: 17–19). Few theological thinkers throughout the early modern period cared to even question the biblical licence to exploit animals. Indeed, the Roman Catholic church appears to have overlooked the issue altogether; perhaps, it has been suggested, because Catholicism assumed there to be a huge gap between animals – that were irrational – and the rational humans who possessed immortal souls (Maehle 1994: 82).

Theological justifications of animal use were further bolstered by philosophical doctrine, as the Cartesian school of thought gained popularity during the seventeenth century. According to Descartes and his followers, animals were simply intricate and soulless machines; automata which, although they could produce apparently complex behaviour, were devoid of the capacity for reason or sensibility. Such thinking provided the legitimisation of much cruelty being inflicted on animals in the name of scientific progress (Serpell 1996; Regan 1983). To what extent both the theological and philosophical thought of the past actually influenced the everyday conduct of ordinary folk towards animals is another matter. Thomas has alluded to many instances of human affection for animals that contradict the view that animals were treated like mechanical objects rather than sentient beings. Moreover, he also reveals that the commitment to the prevailing theological doctrine of human ascendancy may not have always been quite as strong or influential in everyday life as one might be led to believe (Thomas 1983: 92–120).

By the eighteenth century, the bible had become subject to rather less literal interpretation. As a consequence, the notion that humans were the caretakers of the natural world, rather than the controllers of it, grew in popularity and influence. This new-found Christian concept of stewardship entreated that animals should be treated carefully, respectfully and responsibly. Humans had a clear duty to animals to ensure that they were fed, sheltered and cared for adequately, should be slaughtered as quickly and painlessly as possible and not needlessly over-exerted (Maehle 1994: 85). Animals could thus legitimately be exploited for necessary human ends, such as for nourishment and traction, as long as they were exploited with due care and respect. Further to this change in theological thinking, from the mid-eighteenth century onwards, there was increasing interest in the welfare of the animals used by human society, which in turn was supported by a growing knowledge of both animal and human anatomy and physiology which suggested that animals were indeed sentient creatures capable of feeling pain. This issue, with regard to the nature of our use and treatment of animals, came to be encapsulated in Jeremy Bentham's much quoted dictum: 'the question is not, Can they *reason*? Nor, Can they *talk*? But, Can they *suffer*?' (quoted in Regan 1983: 95). Such early discussions on animal sentience and human duties to other creatures provided the basis for the evolution of the animal rights and welfare movements that today either seek to improve the lot of animals in human society or eradicate animal exploitation altogether. Yet, in spite of such changes in thought and theological tradition, as we continue to advance towards the twenty-first century, our use of animals appears to have steadily intensified, rather than to have diminished. As the introductory discussion above demonstrates, it is evident that modern industrial society is highly dependent on the exploitation of animal resources; though, at the same time, we also seem to be far less aware of the great extent of that dependency.

The Christian concept of stewardship and the notion of our duties towards other animals discussed above to some extent touch on the second main theme with which this book is concerned, namely the human responsibility to adequately feed and care for the animals that are used to service human needs. However, when I speak of responsibility, it is not in terms of our duties and moral obligations towards animals, but is instead in terms of human interest. The animals with which this book is primarily concerned are those domesticated species on which we most depend to meet our routine nutritional, economic and affective needs.[3] Most particularly where food-producing animals and beasts of burden are concerned, it has always been in the practical interests of their human owners to ensure that they receive at least the very minimum of nourishment and human attention to their condition. As Andrew Johnson has pointed out, livestock are first and foremost the farmer's property, and must be fed and cared for because of their future value, both monetary and nutritional (Johnson 1991:10). There are, therefore, practical limitations to the way in which animals can be treated. By abusing or neglecting them productivity and profit are potentially put in jeopardy. In order to exploit animals to the full, it is also imperative that they be kept fit and free from disease; otherwise there is a risk that they will fail to adequately fulfil their intended function within human society. By choosing to keep and use other species to meet human needs and requirements, humankind has saddled itself with the responsibility for protecting and preserving their health and well-being: we have, therefore, forced ourselves to endure the burden of beasts.

Animals, Disease and Human Society explores the manner in which people have realised and borne the responsibility for animal health throughout the ages. It tells a tale that begins, some 10,000 years ago, at the point in human history when people first began to incorporate animals within the bounds of human social organisation through the process of domestication. The domestication of animals, I shall argue, has had far-reaching consequences for humankind. Although the enfoldment of animals into human society enabled humans to secure a fairly reliable source of food and other secondary products, it led to an increasing dependence on the social and agricultural arrangements involved in maintaining this resource. Animal domestication and the inception of livestock husbandry, as we shall shortly see, resulted not only in a critical transformation in the relationship between humans and other animals, but also precipitated profound changes in the structure of human society and the nature of social relations. Domesticated animals came to constitute an important natural resource that, although renewable, required careful maintenance. Caring for these animals from the cradle to the table thus became an important preoccupation within human society. People were obliged to develop the practical knowledge, skills and discipline necessary to ensure a continual and healthy supply of food-producing animals. A further and more insidious consequence of animal domestication, and one that is pivotal to this book, was that it created increased opportunities for the transmission of infectious disease. The impact of animal disease on human society is thus a central theme that recurs throughout this book and I have attempted to trace the measures that people have implemented throughout history to reduce or preclude the risks posed by animal disease in order to preserve the health of both human and animal populations.

In this context, I have introduced the concept of the *veterinary regime*. The notion of 'regime' is a particularly useful tool for sociological analysis. In its broadest sense, the term 'regime' may be understood as a 'constellation of more or less institutionalised behaviour' (Spier 1996: 5). It can be seen to neatly encapsulate the complex configurations and interdependency of human relationships, most particularly with respect to the practices and restraints that people (attempt to) impose on each other and on themselves. The concept of regime has in fact enjoyed increasing popularity in the social scientific literature of recent times, particularly in the Netherlands; finding greatest favour among process sociologists, who have, for instance, employed the term in reference to religious regimes, ecological regimes, medical regimes and pedagogical regimes (Spier 1995: 301). Following in their footsteps, I have chosen to employ the term 'veterinary regime' to describe the social practices and institutionalised behaviours that have emerged in response to the problem of maintaining animal resources and protecting human health and economy. This notion is central to my discussion and is intended to epitomise and encapsulate the growing and increasingly formalised ways in which humankind has sought to deal with the problem of animal health and disease as our dependency on animal resources has continued to increase and intensify throughout the course of human history.

This book is, therefore, also one that is very much about the history of animal medicine. It is, however, quite unlike existing attempts to trace the evolution of the veterinary art. Traditionally, accounts of veterinary history (e.g. Smith 1919–33; Smithcors 1957; Karasszon 1988; Pugh 1962; Wester 1939) have tended to focus on the development of the scientific techniques and medical procedures that have furthered the advancement of veterinary medical science throughout the ages. In addition to this, they have also had a tendency to pinpoint and extensively discuss the key figures who have made important contributions to the field of animal medicine. Unfortunately such accounts are often devoid of social context; more to the point, they can often be rather repetitive, caustic in character and, in some instances, have clearly been copied more or less word for word – at least in parts – from earlier sources.[4] Even the most recent – and most beautifully illustrated – publication (Dunlop and Williams 1996) to tell the tale of the history of veterinary medicine has unfortunately fallen foul of adopting this traditional formula. Moreover, even the attempts its authors have made to place the events and developments within a broader cultural, social, economic or political context clearly fall far short of standards of historical adequacy and accuracy; sweeping generalisations and inadequate citation by which one can verify the writers' assertions being perhaps the volume's greatest failings (Koolmees and Mathijsen 1996).

Veterinary history has, as a rule, generally been written by veterinarians interested in, and wishing to generate interest in, the history of their profession, rather than by social historians. For this reason, one can to some extent understand the lack of attention to socio-historical detail and appreciate the fact that veterinary historical authors have often chosen to concentrate exclusively on, for example, the founding and development of veterinary colleges (e.g. Charnock Bradley 1923; Cotchin 1990), the work of military veterinary corps (e.g. Smith 1927), the activities of the overseas veterinary services (e.g. West 1961) or the biography of influential veterinarians (e.g. Pattison 1981, 1990; D'Arcy Thompson 1974). There are, as ever, a few notable exceptions to this rule. In recent years, a handful of authors have succeeded in tackling aspects of veterinary history with a keen eye for historical and cultural detail. For example, Wilkinson (1992) has written extensively on the relationship between animals and disease in her work on the history of comparative medicine; Fisher (1995) analyses the origins of the veterinary profession in Britain, exploring transformations in European culture during the late eighteenth century. Similarly, Offringa (1971, 1976, 1981, 1983) traces the emergence and institutionalisation of the veterinary profession in the Netherlands, drawing on sociological theories of professionalisation to structure his discussion; Koolmees (1997) explores the historical and social changes that underlay the introduction of public slaughterhouses in the Netherlands and the increasingly important role of veterinary meat inspection; and finally, Schwabe (1978) examines early animal medicine and the cattle culture of ancient Sumer and Egypt, employing a considerable amount of comparative anthropological data in his discussion. Of the aforementioned authors, only the latter is in fact a veterinarian; the others are indeed professional historians.

My own account of veterinary history contrasts considerably with existing explorations of the evolution of the veterinary art. It explores how transformations in social relations and the changing interdependencies between humans and other animals were responsible for, or were responses to, the emergence and intensification of the veterinary regime. The technological inventions, medical discoveries, changing surgical procedures or the biographies of individual veterinarians, that have generally been the focus of veterinary history, have thus been of far less interest to me. In this volume, I have attempted to delineate the rise and intensification of the veterinary regime in terms of phases. In short, four successive stages of development of the veterinary regime within European society can be discerned:

1 a stage when there was no (need for any) form of a veterinary regime, either informal or formal;
2 a stage when only an informal veterinary regime existed, but no formal veterinary regime had yet developed;
3 a stage when both an informal and formal veterinary regime coexisted and competed with one another;
4 a stage dominated exclusively by a formal veterinary regime.

This 'phaseology' is largely reflected in the chapter divisions that will shortly be outlined. Exploring the past in terms of phases, or stages of development, is in many respects far more flexible than explaining historical change in terms of specific events and chronology. It is often difficult to say with any great historical precision exactly when or where developments occurred, particularly with respect to the earliest phases in human history. Regarding history in terms of stages of development largely circumvents this problem. This approach to history has in fact been greatly influenced by the work of the Dutch sociologist Johan Goudsblom (1989a, 1992). Goudsblom has convincingly managed to highlight the relevance of history to sociology and has realised the possibilities of employing a long-term sociological perspective. The concept of process that he has introduced provides a most interesting apparatus with which the past can be studied and its relationship to the present understood. It is a dynamic concept that is bound neither by place nor time. Moreover, it allows one to explore history without getting bogged down in a mire of facts, figures, dates and places. Looking at history in terms of social process involves the identification of the major catalysts and trends that have changed the course of human history and have irrevocably transformed the nature of human social life across the globe (Goudsblom 1989a). Goudsblom's work, particularly that on the impact of the domestication of fire on human civilisation, has provided an important model for me both with regard to how a sociologist can approach history and how I should discuss the consequences of animal domestication for human society (Goudsblom 1992). A second major, though related, influence on my discussion of the relationship between animals, disease and human society has been the world historian William H. McNeill. His work, as will become evident in the following chapter, has provided great inspiration for this book. In particular, it was his remarkable work *Plagues and Peoples* (1976) that has acted as a springboard for my own study. In essence, I have attempted to pick up and develop a thread on animal disease and human social life that McNeill briefly introduced in his account of the impact of pestilence on human civilisation.

The theoretical concepts and assumptions that underpin this study are also largely contiguous to my attitude towards history. As my adoption of the term 'regime' suggests, the kind of theoretical approach that I favour owes much to what generally goes under the epithets of figurational or process sociology. This is a brand of sociological analysis that derives from the work of Norbert Elias and his intellectual disciples. At the very core of this theoretical approach lies Elias' magnum opus *The Civilising Process* ([1939]1994). This epic study traces changes in the conduct of the western European upper classes between 1300 and 1800. In sum, Elias argued that these, often subtle, changes in behaviour illuminate the more significant transformation of the structure of society that occurred during this period. According to Elias, the entire personality structure of individuals underwent a significant transformation due to the changes in social relations that occurred alongside the process of state formation and the monopolisation of violence. As people began to exert more subtle constraints on one another, their behavioural patterns and emotional make-up gradually changed, leading to new thresholds in self and social control, in addition to more differentiated patterns of conduct. One of the most significant changes in the personality structure was a growing sensitivity with regard to impulsive violent acts, both in terms of witnessing and committing them. This 'delicacy of feeling', however, extended much further than simply an aversion to brutality and a growing sense of defencelessness. As the chains of interdependence grew and more people were required to live with each other in different ways, sensitivities to other primal aspects of human existence, such as bodily functions and disease, also increased. It is also with this framework in mind that I shall examine the changing nature of relationships between humans and other animals. For example, the increasing concern for animal welfare during the eighteenth century that was mentioned earlier can be viewed as a broader social response to the diminishing contrasts between individuals and increasing sensibilities towards others that were taking place in wider society at that time. Often, in this book, I will discuss the changing interdependencies between humans and other animals; when I do so, Elias' influence should be understood as being implicit to my argument.

Finally, it is pertinent to say a few words about the data on which *Animals, Disease and Human Society* is based. This book is the product of both documentary and ethnographic data that were collected during the course of my doctoral research. During the earliest phase of my inquiries into the nature of the human–animal relationship and veterinary medicine, I spent a considerable amount of time in the company of veterinarians – working in urban, rural and mixed veterinary practices in the Netherlands – as a participant observer. This proved a fascinating experience and afforded me a great deal of insight into the everyday work and social significance of the veterinary profession. Moreover, it also provided me with the opportunity to meet and talk to a wide variety of animal owners and witness the nature of their interactions with their animals, ultimately allowing me to gain a deeper understanding of both people's attachments to other animals (Swabe 1994) and the inherently ambiguous nature of human–animal relations (Swabe 1996). Accompanying vets also granted me access to particular settings – namely the farms where livestock are intensively produced – where I would otherwise most likely not have been particularly welcome. Further to this, watching veterinarians at work also helped rid me of many of my preconceptions and romantic illusions about what vets do. Within a short space of time, it became clear that veterinary heroics, such as saving dying or injured animals, played a fairly limited role in daily veterinary practice, whereas tasks such as inoculation, parasite control, blood testing and neutering took up most of the average veterinarian's time. As a consequence of these observations, my focus shifted decisively from looking at the curative to the preventative nature of veterinary work, in addition to the role that veterinarians play in the management of animal (re)production.

In the course of my research, my project gained an increasingly historical character, eventually leading to the painful conclusion that much of the fascinating data I had collected in these early stages would, by necessity, have to be omitted from the end product. However, at times it will be evident, particularly in the latter chapters that deal with the twentieth century, that my discussion is based in part on my own experiences and direct observations of veterinary work. In contrast to my ethnographic research, the gathering of historical data chiefly involved tracking down as wide a variety of primary literary sources – or translations thereof – as possible, dating from classical times up until the present day, in order to learn more about the rise of the veterinary regime. Doing so proved most worthwhile, for much of the literature that I studied – particularly the material dating from the seventeenth, eighteenth and nineteenth centuries – often turned out to be replete with social rhetoric and historical detail that has generally been omitted from existing historical accounts of veterinary literature and ideas on animal medicine. Wherever possible, I have attempted to refer to such primary data, rather than depending on secondary sources. In addition to these ethnographic and historical documentary sources, being a truly 'free-range' researcher, I have also gleaned data from informal interviews with veterinary professionals and a wide variety of other information reservoirs such as newspapers, television documentaries and the Internet.

An outline of the book

As the above discussion has already indicated, this book traces changes in the human–animal relationship and the rise of the veterinary regime from the time of animal domestication and the inception of livestock husbandry up until the present day. The book, therefore, has an enormous scope and encompasses a huge time-span. My discussion is often at the level of the general, rather than the specific. I have no pretensions to have written a concise and complete history of human–animal relations and animal medicine; that certainly has not been the object of the exercise. My intention is to give the reader an impression and understanding of changing human relations and the long-term and far-reaching consequences thereof for human society. As my discussion moves through time, it will become increasingly more specific and directed to the developments that have occurred within European society. One could thus see my discussion as a funnel that starts at the broadest level some 10,000 years ago with the origins of agriculture and animal domestication and gradually narrows down to focus on developments that occurred in Europe in recent centuries. In particular, many of the examples that are given derive specifically from Britain and the Netherlands; this is largely due to the limitations of language and the practical constraints of research. Particularly where developments in veterinary medicine are concerned, both the British and Dutch examples are indeed somewhat quirky. Yet, as will become evident later in this volume, they provide an exceptionally good illustration of the necessity for the development of an effective state-directed veterinary regime – as to some extent already existed in other parts of western Europe during the nineteenth century – and the consequences of failing to do so.

Leaving such issues aside, I shall now briefly outline the content and structure of this book. As a whole, the book is structured in a 'phaseological' and thematic fashion. The following chapter begins with an examination of animal domestication and the origins of agriculture, and explores the consequences of these developments in terms of human social relations and infectious disease. More importantly, this chapter also sets out the main theoretical model – on the relationship between our control of, dependency on and vulnerability to animals – which will be returned to, both explicitly and implicitly, throughout the whole book. Chapter 3 seeks to explore the relationship between animals, disease and human society from ancient times up until the early modern period. It will discuss the increasing exploitation of animals and the nature of human–animal interdependence within agrarian society, with specific emphasis on the effects of epidemics and epizootics on the agricultural economy. This chapter will also examine the character of early animal medicine and notions on animal disease and its control.

Chapter 4 is concerned with the impact of the transition from agrarianism to industrialisation on the nature of human–animal relations and animal medicine. It explores how the scientific enlightenment, urbanisation and the changing nature of social relations influenced the establishment of formal veterinary education, heralding the birth of the veterinary profession in Europe. This chapter thus looks at the gradual formalisation and intensification of the veterinary regime. In this regard, it also examines the emergent role of the state in dealing with the epizootic disease that plagued the nations of Europe during the early industrial age. Governmental responses to outbreaks of cattle plague in Britain and the Netherlands during the nineteenth century will form the basis of the discussion. Chapter 5 continues this tale of state intervention and control into the twentieth century. This chapter explores the rapid intensification of livestock production during this century and the consequent further intensification of the veterinary regime. It examines the increasing risks to animal welfare, health and environment that the increased exploitation of animal resources has posed, discussing the increasingly important role of the state and the internationalisation of animal disease control. Further to this, this chapter examines the role of the individual large-animal veterinary practitioner in the maintenance and preservation of both animal and public health.

Chapter 6 explores the nature and history of our relationship with the animals that we keep as pets, rather than those on which we depend for food. It looks at our increasing intimacy with and affective dependency on small animals, and explores how the veterinary regime has been extended since the mid-nineteenth century to encompass and care for pet animals. The theme of animal disease and public health will also recur in this chapter in the light of a consideration of the health benefits and drawbacks of keeping animals as pets. Lastly, Chapter 7 attempts to bring together and recapitulate the main themes discussed in the volume and will consider what the future holds for the human–animal relationship. Chapter 7 thus explores recent biotechnological advances, such as the genetic modification and cloning of animals, and discusses the newly emerging possibilities for the increased exploitation of animals, e.g. xenotransplantation, the production of biopharmaceuticals, etc., that are on today's scientific agenda. The genetic modification of animals will be considered not only as a novel form of animal exploitation, but will also be taken to epitomise humankind's increasing dependence on animals as a resource. The consequences of such developments will also be discussed in terms of disease, human health and the implications for the future role of veterinary medical science in society.

2

DOMESTICATION, DEPENDENCY AND DISEASE

Introduction

The most primal relationship between humans and other animals is that of predator and prey. The necessity to eat and avoid being eaten characterises the quest for survival in which both humans and other animals have been engaged throughout the course of evolution. As they evolved, humans became increasingly more formidable predators, capable of securing sustenance not only through consuming plant foods, but also by eating animal protein. Animal flesh was at first most likely procured by scavenging on the remains of creatures, which had either been felled by other predators, or had died a natural death. In time, hominids and their archaic human successors became skilled predators. Freshly killed animals were consumed for food, their skins used to provide warmth, their bones as the raw materials for tools and their marrow eaten for extra sustenance. Nevertheless, in spite of their hunting prowess, meat probably played only a secondary role in our ancestors' diet. Even after they had become accomplished predators, the bulk of their nourishment was most likely derived from plant sources, insects, grubs and birds' eggs. However, irrespective of the quantity or frequency of meat consumption, feasting on the carcasses of dead animals – whether deliberately killed or simply scavenged on – had potentially grave consequences for humans. Eating meat, particularly when raw or poorly cooked, could result in illness and mortality.[1]

Although humans became accomplished hunters, the prey that they stood the greatest chance of killing and consuming were inevitably the old, diseased or crippled animals, or the very young. Healthier adult animals would have been more able to successfully flee from their predators (Baker and Brothwell 1980: 2). If, however, an animal was diseased, infection could potentially be transmitted to humans through its flesh, marrow, and possibly even its skin. It is, for example, likely that during the Pleistocene era cattle herds were affected by tuberculosis. The ingestion of meat contaminated by bovine tuberculosis bacteria would have resulted in the possible transfer of infection to humans, who if affected by the bacteria stood the chance of developing serious illness. The weakest and most poorly nourished people would probably have been most seriously affected, whereas the more robust might have only developed mild or no symptoms whatsoever (Manchester 1984: 162–3). Similarly, animals afflicted with other internal parasitic diseases might have caused humans to become ill if their flesh was ingested. For instance, protozoal infections, such as toxoplasmosis, could have been passed to humans from their prey (Brothwell 1991: 19). It is also probable that tapeworms blighted our ancestors. They too would have been acquired through ingestion in their larval form in the flesh of pigs, cattle and other herbivores. Like their animal and human hosts, such parasites are thought to have a long evolutionary history. It has, for instance, been suggested that the cysticercus larvae responsible for causing tapeworm infestation in humans originated long before *Homo sapiens* emerged (Fiennes 1978: 12). In addition to this, tick-borne infections, such as tularaemia, would probably have been associated with increased prowess in hunting and a closer relationship with prey, e.g. meat processing and skin preparation (Brothwell 1991: 19).

In the case of some of these internal conditions it might not have been immediately obvious that the animal's flesh was tainted. More apparent imperfections such as external lesions, particularly those exuding pus, would probably not have been consumed. Suppurating flesh was most likely cut away and discarded (Baker and Brothwell 1980: 2). Likewise, putrefying animal flesh would probably have been avoided. The consumption of rotten meat potentially leads to stomach upsets, if not more serious complaints, and it would doubtless not have taken our ancestors long to associate their illness with what they had recently eaten. In terms of physical development and brain size, our Palaeolithic ancestors differed very little from humans today. One can therefore presume that they had sufficient mental capacity to ascertain which foodstuffs were liable to cause illness and to transmit this knowledge culturally. Moreover, it is conceivable that early humans developed an elementary understanding of meat hygiene and animal disorders. Archaeological analyses of food bone debris, dating from the late Pleistocene, evidence butchery marks, which indicate complex forms of meat processing (Brothwell 1991).

The religious practices of ancient civilisations and modern hunter-gatherers, particularly with regard to sacrifice and food taboos, suggest that early meat hygiene – if it existed – would have been tied to spiritual beliefs and ritual. Notions of purity and defilement probably led not only to a reluctance to eat the flesh of animals that had not deliberately been slaughtered, but to bloodshed becoming of central value to meat itself. Meat from animals that had not died by the human hand belongs to the category of the unknown and was, therefore, probably not eaten (Fiddes 1991: 65). In ancient cultures, religious decrees ordained that animals chosen for sacrifice must be flawless. Offering diseased or disfigured animals to the gods would incite their wrath. Furthermore, if the flesh of such animals was eaten, it was thought that humans might be cursed with disease (Koolmees 1991: 9). Similar beliefs may have influenced early human societies in their selection of meat for human consumption and the development of rudimentary standards of meat hygiene.

Apart from the potential for contamination with disease through meat consumption, procuring animal flesh might have presented other risks to life and limb for our ancestors. The more advanced and organised forms of hunting, such as game drives, entailed a risk of being trampled to death or mortally wounded, particularly if animals behaved unpredictably. Skeletal remains suggest that our Palaeolithic ancestors were considerably smaller than us. The ungulate species on which they preyed, however, were substantially larger and undoubtedly less placid than their domesticated descendants. For instance, the aurochs, the progenitor of domestic cattle, stood at least two metres at the shoulder, with long menacing horns and probably a temperament to match (Clutton-Brock 1987: 64). These enormous beasts were likely to have inflicted fatal injury on any human that stood in their path. By the same token, encounters with humans most likely had similar consequences for animals. Injuries sustained by animals in flight of their human predators or from projectiles hurled at them would most certainly have weakened them leading eventually to death, or increased susceptibility to other adversaries. Our ancestors, if unfortunate, were the quarry of other large animals. The archaic human body was doubtless host to numerous parasitic infestations, which would have been deleterious to the health of any predator that consumed its flesh. Cadavers of humans who died a natural death – and were neither buried nor burned – would also have provided carnivorous scavengers with both a convenient supply of meat and a possible source of infection.

Food thus formed the fundamental basis for the earliest interactions between humans and other animal species. In essence, food is a central problem of ecology. In principle, the natural world lives in balance, albeit often an uneasy one. The concept of the food chain neatly encapsulates the nature and complexity of the web of interdependencies and symbioses between species. One species will prey on another which in turn will provide nourishment for yet another and so forth. This predatory relationship is often explicit; the animal that eats will be larger or stronger than the one that is eaten. However, even when a species appears immune to outside attack, it is inevitably vulnerable to attack from within. The enemy may be invisible to the naked eye, parasitically living within or feeding on the tissue of the apparently invulnerable, either directly or through an intermediary such as an insect. As Burnet and White observe, 'the tiger may be lord of the jungle, but its lungs may be riddled with parasitic worms' (Burnet and White 1972: 7). Microparasites operate more or less like other predators – one simply cannot see them with the naked eye. Microbes are omnipresent where any other living creature exists and play an important role for all life on Earth. The vast majority of microorganisms which live in animals, including humans, are either commensal or perform a valuable function within the animal host. They are perfectly adapted to and live harmlessly in symbiosis with their hosts. Microbes, for instance, help their host to digest and gain nutrients from food. They can, however, as the above discussion suggests, have a detrimental effect on their animal hosts, or on the predators who eat them. In short, microorganisms can cause disease.

Disease occurs as the consequence of a microbe entering a host, or part of a host, to which it is not wholly adapted, but within which it can grow and flourish. As a result of this incursion, the host's biological defences are brought into action. If these defensive processes are overtaxed or unsuccessful, the host becomes ill and may die. If the host expires, the parasitic organism will perish, since it is deprived of a living host on which it can feed. That is, of course, unless it can find a new one. The parasites which are poorly adapted to the host, or accidentally find themselves in a new host, are thus the most dangerous and potentially lethal (Postgate 1992: 51–3). There are many ways in which pathogenic organisms can be transmitted to their new host. As illustrated above, our ancestors were most likely blighted by disease-causing organisms that they ingested along with the flesh of their animal prey. Pathogens, however, can also be transmitted by droplet infection, in soil or water, through the exchange of bodily fluids and the bite or incursion of an intermediate host, such as an insect. The balance between parasite and host can thus be disturbed leading to potentially devastating consequences for either one or both parties. Likewise, the equilibrium between predator and prey can be destabilised, leading to profound repercussions for the entire ecological system – including the relationship between microparasites and their hosts.

This chapter is concerned with the changing relationship between human predators and their animal prey and its impact on natural ecological balances. Human evolutionary success, cultural development and expansion into new environmental realms led to fundamental changes in the relationship between species. The gradual shift from hunting animals to herding them, which began within some human societies around 10,000 years ago, transformed the age-old relationship between human predator and animal prey forever. Rather than devoting their attention merely to procuring meat and other by-products of dead animals, some human groups began to turn their attention to living animals in a bid to obtain their nourishment (Meadow 1989). The emergence of agriculture and animal husbandry not only had significant consequences for the further course of human–animal relations, but it also had a profound impact on the way in which human beings lived together. Furthermore, the ecological transformation exacted by the shift to an agrarian regime led to the irreversible disruption of delicate ecological balances, creating new and potentially lethal threats to the health and well-being of humankind and that of other animals. In this chapter, I will explore the consequences of animal domestication and agrarianisation for the human–animal relationship, human social life and health. First, however, I shall examine the sociocultural evolution of humankind, which eventually culminated in domestication, and the establishment of an agrarian regime. There have, in recent times, been numerous attempts to explain why – after many thousands of years – our ancestors abandoned scavenging, hunting and gathering in favour of animal husbandry and agriculture. In this chapter, I have chosen to outline some of the most influential and interesting of these theories. By producing such a synthesis of recent thought on the origins of agriculture and animal domestication, I hope to paint a backdrop for my own story, which is, in essence, a tale of domestication, dependency and disease.

The origins of agriculture: the changing human relationship with the natural world

The detail that we possess on early human social life and cultural development, prior to the emergence of written records, is derived largely from the analysis of fragments excavated from our remote past. Geological conditions, geographical location and carbon-dating can help us to locate archaeological artefacts in place and time. Objects such as animal bones – crucial to understanding domestication – yield fragments of information about the occurrence and morphology of particular animals, the climate and environment in which they lived and even the diseases or injuries from which they suffered. They can also indirectly suggest the existence of a broad range of human activities such as hunting, butchery, agriculture, trade and even religion. Marks on bone fragments, for example, may indicate whether an animal was skinned, chopped up or its flesh cooked. Moreover, it can be deduced what kind of implements were used to prepare the carcass. Similarly, dental wear might indicate that an animal wore a bit and was harnessed. In this way, it can be determined where, when and which human groups exploited animals for traction or transport (Rackham 1994: 14–15). In addition to the analysis and comparison of such archaeological artefacts, the detail of the past is filled in through extrapolation from both anthropological studies of present-day hunter-gatherers and ethological data.

From all these data, it is possible to reconstruct the past. The knowledge that has been gleaned from archaeological artefacts and objects is, however, in itself the source of contention amongst experts. The past is continually being reinterpreted in the light of new findings and theories about our ancestors and the way in which they lived. What is clear, though, is that the emergence of humankind and its various exploits are, in terms of the history of the Earth as a whole, very recent developments. As Marvin Harris succinctly puts it, 'if the evolutionary clock from the origin of life to the present is reduced to the scale of 1 year, human beings make their appearance at about 8 p.m. on New Year's Eve' (Harris 1985b: 42). The recentness of the processes of domestication and agrarianisation can be put into even greater perspective when they are situated within the broader context of millions of years of hominid and human evolution. The first true hominids emerged some five million years ago; being followed a couple of million years later by *Homo sapiens.* Hominids and archaic humans, however, spent the best part of their existence as scavengers, foragers, hunters and gatherers. It was only a mere 10,000 years ago that some, but by no means all, of our ancestors took the first tentative steps towards domestication, animal husbandry and the cultivation of plants: these activities in fact account for less than one per cent of hominid existence (Davis 1987: 126).

Domestication is generally taken to be the historical milestone that marks the most profound and definitive transformation in the relationship between humans and other species. Domestication is not only seen to symbolise the critical transition from simply taking from nature to actively controlling it, but is also generally taken to represent the move which most clearly distinguished humans from other animals. Yet although food production through animal and plant husbandry is a development which very clearly separated human beings from other animals, the differentiation between humans and other species began to take shape long before humans switched from hunting animals to herding them. Domestication was far from an overnight occurrence. On the contrary, it was a gradual process which in fact continues to the present day, subtly altering the behaviour, appearance, functioning and distribution of other species and, consequently, our relationship to them. In the following discussion, I will explore the development of humankind and its changing relationship with other species. It will become clear that as our own species developed into proficient formidable hunters and then agriculturalists, the balance of power between humans and other animals gradually shifted in favour of humans. The balance of power between humans and microparasites, however, is another matter entirely, which will be dealt with later.

The gradual differentiation of behaviour and power between humans and other animals can be traced alongside the gradual biological and socio-cultural development of humankind. The biological evolution of humankind led to the emergence of distinctive physiological traits such as an erect posture, dextrous hands, a highly developed brain and the capacity to communicate through the use of symbols and facial expression. The latter two characteristics ultimately gave rise to the development of the complex patterns of cultural transmission and social organisation that are peculiar to humankind (Goudsblom 1990). The earliest cultural innovation which our ancestors made was probably the manufacture and use of tools. The most primitive stone tools unearthed by archaeologists date back around 2.5 million years. Although such tools offer us some material evidence of culture, they do not necessarily indicate the degree of cultural sophistication their manufacturers possessed (Ucko and Dimbleby 1969). Moreover, given the ability of other primates, most particularly chimpanzees, to use objects taken from their immediate surrounds as tools, we must be cautious as to the importance we place on such developments in relation to how they distinguished our forebears from other species.

The innovation that fundamentally and decisively separated our hominid ancestors from other animal species was the mastery of fire. The domestication of fire provides the most tangible testimony to human cultural influence on ecological processes. Archaeological evidence suggests that our predecessors *Homo erectus* were actively manipulating this natural phenomenon some 400,000 years ago. How efficient these hominids were at using this resource is here not the issue. Suffice it to say that over the course of time, these hominids and then their more successful successors – archaic humans – developed the mental, physical and social skills necessary to keep fires burning and to actively use fire to protect themselves. As Goudsblom (1990, 1992) argues, the ability to control and reproduce this natural force and use it to their advantage effectively allowed our ancestors to gain a degree of superiority over the other species with whom they were competing for food. Notwithstanding the complex cultural transmission, foresight and self-constraint necessary to achieve and maintain the control of fire, early humans – through their singular and eventually universal ability to manipulate this natural substance – ensured their own species' survival above that of their predatory competitors. Fire control enabled human populations to move north to explore new territories and to survive the cold glacial climates of the Ice Age. Furthermore, it extended the variety and availability of animal foods, since meat could not only be cooked, but could also be preserved through smoking or drying (Clutton-Brock 1987: 188). In short, by mastering fire, humans clearly distinguished themselves from other animals and improved their survival chances and predatory skill. Moreover, as a consequence of fire domestication, the fates of other species – both animal and plant – were to be inextricably linked with human evolution and socio-cultural development.

The gradual social and cultural evolution of humankind laid the foundations for the eventual domestication of animals and plants. Alongside the socio-cultural developments which accompanied tool and fire use, our progenitors achieved a high degree of social organisation through their hunting activities. It has been suggested that the hunting of large ungulates during the Pleistocene period was probably 'one of the formative activities that led to the integration and coordination of all other behavioural patterns in the social evolution of humans' (Clutton-Brock 1994: 24). Human predatory success is most closely linked to our species' highly social nature. The need to provide food for the collective plausibly formed the basis for the exceptionally complex social behaviour of human beings. Although other social carnivores such as wolves were probably as effective group predators as humans, our ancestors were able to surpass them through both a high degree of cooperation between individuals and the development of increasingly innovative means of killing animals, such as the use of projectiles and setting fire to forests in order to drive animal herds to their deaths (Clutton-Brock 1994: 24). In addition to this, a detailed knowledge and understanding of the behaviour of other animals would have been imperative to the successful hunting of them. The recognition of changing seasons, the migration patterns of animal herds, seasonal appearance of various plants and flowers, and knowing which parts of animals and plants were good to eat, etc., facilitated human survival, for such environmental appreciation – and the cultural transmission thereof – would have provided our forebears with constant and varying sources of nourishment.

Humans, in short, became highly efficient hunters and gatherers, capable of finding sustenance under whatever circumstances, both climatic and geographic, they found themselves. This manner of subsistence continued unabated for many thousands of years of human existence. Our ancestors lived an exclusively nomadic life, surviving by moving from place to place searching for, or following, potential prey and accumulating fresh stocks of plant food. However, around ten thousand years ago, a fundamental and irreversible change in human lifestyle was initiated. Some human groups began to settle, and the hunter-gatherer way of life was gradually supplanted by the tending of livestock and the tilling of land. Just why some of our forebears forsook the ways of old for an inherently more arduous and precarious existence is unclear. It is generally acknowledged that there must have been some kind of environmental pressure that forced them to tend their quarry rather than track it. Numerous hypotheses – often explicitly based on Malthusian principles of causality – have been put forward to explain this transition. The most renowned theory on the origins of agriculture was advanced by the archaeologist V. Gordon Childe during the 1930s. It was in fact Childe who coined the expression 'the Neolithic Revolution'. He believed that this phrase would highlight the inception of agriculture as a crucial stage of human cultural development – a great, though not sudden, leap forward for humankind. In Childe's view, the substantial reorganisation of technology, which the emergence of agriculture involved over a relatively short period of time, resulted in periods of rapid population growth and the reorganisation of social institutions (Cohen 1977: 2–3). Domestication, he argued, occurred as a consequence of post-glacial desiccation. Childe postulated that after the last Ice Age, regions such as the Near East became far drier. Shrinking water sources meant that the environment could no longer support as much animal life as previously. This led to the concentration of populations around fertile oases, subsequently forcing humans and other animals into developing intimate and mutually dependent relations. Rather than parasitically taking from nature, Childe argued, Neolithic societies began to cooperate with it to protect and increase the productivity of plants and other animals (Ucko and Dimbleby 1969; Barker 1985; Redman 1978).

More recent research has cast considerable doubt on whether such drought and the creation of oases actually occurred at the end of the Pleistocene (Cohen 1977: 8). Since Childe, many hypotheses have been put forward to explain the origins of agriculture. Some of these have focused on the cultural conditions, suggesting that sedentism and the consequent intimacy and familiarity with flora and fauna led to domestication. Other theories contend that the shift to agriculture was precipitated by population pressure. During the 1960s, for instance, the economist Ester Boserup stressed that population pressure results in imbalances in resources which in turn leads to the adoption of organised food production – the most intensive kind of subsistence strategy of all. Increasingly productive methods of agriculture, she argued, demand increasingly more time and energy on the part of food producers. The agricultural mode of food production would thus only have been adopted as a result of the population pressures caused by extensive growth in areas which are unable to sustain such high levels of exploitation (Barker 1985: 8). In a similar vein, Mark Cohen (1977) has developed an elaborate population pressure model to explain the origins of agriculture. Cohen explained domestication as a necessary and intentional adaptation, which occurred to meet the imminent crisis presented by overpopulation, increasing human food needs, and the failure of the natural environment to produce enough to satisfy them. The coincidence of increased population pressure and significant climatic changes following the last Ice Age, he argues, resulted in the decline of environmental productivity and a reduction in the nutritional adequacy of the human diet, leading first to the deliberate cultivation of crops and subsequently to the subjugation of animals, particularly in the Near East. Cohen's theory, albeit persuasive, has also come under fire. More recent archaeological analysis of human remains dating from the period just prior to the dawn of agriculture shows no evidence of malnutrition, thus contradicting his theory (Cohen and Armelagos 1984: 597).

In addition to the above explanations, there exist less well-known hypotheses about the origins of agriculture which are, perhaps, less easily verifiable through the examination of archaeological artefacts. Hayden (1992), for example, has submitted an alternative explanation for the transition to agriculture, which, he argues, does not hinge on notions of population pressure, climatic change or 'other relatively popular explanatory factors' (Hayden 1992: 11). Instead he proposes a 'competitive feasting' model to explain the domestication of plants and animals. Hayden suggests that population levels in hunter-gatherer societies are maintained in dynamic equilibrium with available food resources. Such societies necessarily operate on the basis of food sharing since they are dependent on unpredictable resources that can easily be over-exploited. The obligatory sharing of food, he argues, makes any labour investment in producing food pointless. Everyone has equal access to food and, when resources are low, the entire group simply moves elsewhere to where it is more plentiful (Hayden 1992: 12). According to Hayden, the shift to agricultural food production could only occur in the more technologically complex hunter-gatherer societies where fundamental resources were reliably found in abundance and were invulnerable to over-exploitation. Under these circumstances, people could survive without being obliged to share food with one another. Domestication therefore, according to this view, occurred initially in the areas of abundant resources. The first species to be domesticated, he contends, were not used to provide dietary staples; they were instead used to produce delicacies, most specifically for competitive feasts. Drawing on ethnographic evidence, Hayden asserts that such feasts emerged as a result of the establishment of more defined social hierarchies. Ambitious individuals would demonstrate their power and success by being able to produce such luxury foods through intensive production. Domesticated food, he argued, would only be depended on as staples once they could be produced competitively with other available food resources, e.g. wild game (Hayden 1992: 12–13). This novel theory clearly challenges the idea that agricultural production emerged in response to scarcity. However, one could conversely explain such feasting as a ritual recognition of the importance of specific animal species to a particular society and that society's dependence on them. Such ceremonial feasting and ritual sacrifice may, therefore, have had a disciplinary function, to teach people not to kill animals indiscriminately, thereby conserving an important resource (Goudsblom 1989b).

In recent years, explanations of the origins of agriculture and domestication have tended to move away from theorising about human innovative response to environmental change or speculating about early human social relations. Instead these developments have been increasingly viewed as the product of evolutionary process (e.g. Rindos 1984; Budiansky 1992). This approach will be discussed below with respect to the domestication process specifically. Whatever the possible environmental, socio-economic or evolutionary reasons for the switch to agriculture, there is a general consensus that the first synchronous steps towards domestication were made in the Near East and east Asia. A separate, probably later, centre of domestication has been located in the Americas, particularly around Mexico and the Andes. Since the end of the nineteenth century, the Near East has been portrayed as the 'hearth of agriculture' and it is here that evidence of early human settlement and the remains of the progenitors of our most important domestic livestock species, i.e. sheep, goats, cattle and pigs, have been unearthed (Davis 1987: 128). It is thought that during the early Holocene (i.e. the period extending from 10,000 years ago to the present day), this arid region – often described as the 'fertile crescent' – had insufficient natural resources to sustain the growing human population. This was in contrast to the colder northern and western Europe, where large mammals such as deer still lived in abundance and wild nuts provided bountiful plant foods, allowing human populations to continue leading a hunter-gatherer existence (Clutton-Brock 1987: 47–8). However, for humans to survive in the warmer Near East, it became necessary to store food in order to endure times of scarcity. The extreme temperatures experienced in this region make the preservation of animal flesh more problematic than in colder, northern climates. Under such conditions, meat rots quickly, even when dried, rendering it unpleasant to eat if not deleterious to one's health. The establishment of grain reservoirs, supplemented by the storage of meat in the form of livestock, would not only have provided a more palatable and healthy supply of animal protein, but would have extended the possible range of human settlement in this region (Clutton-Brock 1994: 25–6).

It has in fact been suggested that the deliberate cultivation of plants not only preceded animal domestication, but was also an important factor that gave rise to it. As humans began to settle and produce grain, the herds of wild sheep and goats, which naturally fed on wild grasses, were forced into closer proximity to humans in their search for food. This, of course, would have made hunting far easier; people would not have to go in search of their prey, instead it would more or less come to them. However, the movement of these flocks would have to be restricted – most probably with the aid of dogs – in order to stop them consuming the best of the grain, and their numbers could be artificially controlled by slaughtering male animals to conserve both the species and the crops (Harris 1985b: 157–8). Because human movements were limited by settlement and crop cultivation, there was a great danger that over-hunting would greatly reduce the supply of animal protein and hide, possibly leading to the extinction of species. Keeping and maintaining animals as livestock would thus ensure the local availability and a renewable supply of meat. Zeuner (1963) also viewed the domestication of animals as a necessary development to prevent 'crop-robbing' herbivores such as cattle from devouring human crops and depleting the grain supplies necessary to survive the winter. As a corollary to this, Clutton-Brock has suggested that the need to keep marauding animals away from growing crops might have also provided the incentive for early agriculturalists to keep tethered goats or sheep as a 'live store of meat' (Clutton-Brock 1994: 26).

Animal domestication

Domestication is most commonly portrayed as a fundamental change in the nature of the human–animal relationship. Some authors have envisaged domestication more as a continuation of existing human–animal relations; in other words, as an extension or elaboration of the hunter–prey relationship, rather than as a complete break from it. Domestication can in this way be viewed as the end product of a series of gradually intensifying relationships between humans and other animals (Higgs and Jarman 1969). With respect to this, Jarman and Wilkinson (1972) deem it inappropriate to focus merely on the dichotomy between the wild and the domestic. They suggest that this represents only one aspect of a wide range of close relationships between humans and other animals. Marginal cases, such as the reindeer economies and game-cropping of the present day, they argue, imply that this dichotomy may not have been so clear cut in the distant past (Jarman and Wilkinson 1972: 83). Similarly, Hecker has proposed a broad spectrum of human–animal interactions, ranging from the cooperative driving of animals to specialised hunting and culling to finally the selective breeding of domestic livestock (Hecker 1982: 220–3). Although this view of domestication highlights varying degrees of cultural manipulation and control which evolved over time to obtain animal protein, it fails to fully account for the radical changes in human social life and behaviour that animal domestication brought with it in its wake. As Bökönyi points out, although human activities have – in some way or another – always interfered with the lives of other animals, domestication is 'an interference of a quite different kind' (Bökönyi 1969: 219).

The profound social significance of the transition from hunting to herding has, however, been incorporated into several recent definitions of domestication. Meadow, for example, describes animal domestication as being a 'selective diachronic process of change in human–animal relationships involving, at the very least, a change in focus on the part of humans from the dead to the living animal and, more particularly, from the dead animal to the principal product of the living animal – its progeny' (Meadow 1989: 81). This process, he argues, manifests itself in two respects: first, in terms of the transformations in the social and economic structure of the human societies which associate with the animals; and secondly, in the behavioural, morphological and physiological changes which the animal undergoes as a consequence of domestication (Meadow ibid.). Similarly, Clutton-Brock defines a domesticated animal as 'one that has been bred in captivity for purposes of economic profit to a human community that maintains complete mastery over its breeding, organisation of territory, and food supply' (Clutton-Brock 1987: 21). She goes on to argue that domestication is both a cultural and biological process which 'can only take place when tamed animals are incorporated into the social structure of the human group and become objects of ownership'. The morphological transformation of the animal occurs subsequent to its initial integration into human society (Clutton-Brock 1989: 7).

The successful domestication of animals was most likely the product of a long-term process of trial and error. It has been suggested that early human efforts to tame other animals were a product of the highly social nature of humankind. Clutton-Brock, for instance, contends that the enfoldment of other species into human society was an extension of the practices of 'sharing, nurturing and protecting weaker members of the human group' (Clutton-Brock 1994: 24). The assumption that our ancestors would have been prepared to tolerate or support weaker persons, other than perhaps infants and young children, let alone members of other species, is somewhat suspect. Historical and anthropological accounts, however, confirm that in some societies, women suckled young mammals along with their human offspring (Serpell 1989, 1996; Clutton-Brock 1987, 1994). This suggests that within early hunting and gathering societies, juvenile animals were perhaps trapped, nurtured and raised alongside humans and were granted a certain level of protection by their human captors. The European explorers of the eighteenth and nineteenth centuries recorded many instances of pet-keeping and affection for small animals amongst the indigenous peoples they encountered. On the basis of their accounts, during the late nineteenth century, Francis Galton postulated that the 'savage' penchant for taming and caring for small animals as pets provided the basis for the development of livestock keeping (Serpell 1989: 10).

This notion has in fact provided a cornerstone for many explanations of the origins of domestication, most particularly with regard to the early assimilation of dogs into human society. Archaeological findings suggest that *Canis familiaris* was probably the first animal species to undergo domestication. Unlike later domesticates, dogs were not – as far as we are aware – much eaten. Instead, they were most likely used as an aid for obtaining meat. It is widely assumed that the domestic dog descends directly from wolves. Wolves exhibit complex social behavioural patterns similar to humans. They are efficient group predators with a social structure based on a dominance hierarchy. It is thought that our ancestors began to develop a close association with wolves by rearing young cubs that they had caught or found. The hypothesis follows that some of the more placid of these animals reached maturity and accepted human beings as pack members in their adulthood. These tamed animals began to breed in human captivity and, over several generations, eventually developed behavioural characteristics distinct from their wild relatives. This process ultimately culminated in the evolution of a separate kind of animal: the dog (Clutton-Brock 1987: 34–8). Humans and wolves were probably close competitors for food. They shared the same prey and it is likely that they came into close contact, wolves possibly learning to scavenge on the leftovers from human game drives and the parts of animals which humans preferred not to eat in times of plenty (Hyams 1972: 7–8). Although one can speculate on a mutual interest in proximity, it is perhaps more probable that humans saw a way of surpassing their lupine competitors in predation and securing food for themselves by using tamed adult wolves – and eventually dogs – to help in the hunt by detecting and tracking game, and later to help herd other animals rather than prey on them (Clutton-Brock 1994: 25).

The dog is unique amongst early domesticates, given that it was probably not domesticated specifically for food. Most species that underwent domestication were probably intended as 'walking larders'. Sheep, goats and cattle, for example, were most likely exploited as transportable sources of meat and other animal by-products. At a later stage, as we shall see in the following chapter, species such as the horse, donkey and camel were domesticated to provide muscle power for transport and traction, although their meat and milk were also consumed long before they began to perform these roles in human society. Although humankind was effectively able to secure a constant supply of animal protein for itself through the enfoldment of animals into human society, the fact remains that only a handful of species were ever domesticated successfully. As Table 1 illustrates, there are comparatively few domesticated species commonly found in Europe today.[2] The majority of these species originated in the Near East; others descend from the Americas and were only introduced to the European continent following the discovery of the New World. Whilst the appearance and behaviour of these species have changed dramatically since their incorporation into human society, they have flourished under human protection and have, in some instances, outlived their wild or ancestral counterparts. However, as Clutton-Brock points out, the benefits of living under the umbrella of human protection are somewhat dubious. Despite the massive population size and geographic distribution of domesticated animal species in contrast to their wild progenitors, these species have suffered 'irretrievable loss of genetic diversity and evolutionary autonomy' (Clutton-Brock 1994: 27).

Although one might convincingly argue that this small number of species has adequately met the needs and requirements of human society, both past and present, it is nonetheless surprising that so few species were actually domesticated by our ancestors. Historical accounts confirm that other animal species such as the oryx and hyaena were successfully tamed in ancient times, yet these species

Table 1 Domesticated species commonly found in modern Europe, their probable wild ancestors, region and approximate date of earliest domestication

Species of Animal	*Wild Ancestor*	*Region of Origin*	*Approximate Date*
Dog	Wolf	Near East	10,000 BC
Sheep	Asiatic mouflon	Near East	7000 BC
Goat	Bezoar goat	Near East	7000 BC
Cattle	Aurochs	Near East	6000+BC
Pig	Wild boar	Near East	6000+BC
Donkey	Wild ass	Near East	3500 BC
Horse	Tarpan	southern Russia	4000 BC
Cat	Wild cat	Near East	6000 BC
Ferret	Western polecat	NW Africa/Iberia	?
Guinea-pig	Cavy	Peru	? 5000–1000 BC
Rabbit	Wild rabbit	Iberia	? 1000 BC
Chicken	Red jungle fowl	India–Burma	? 2000 BC
Turkey	Wild turkey	Mexico	?

Source: Davis (1987).

were never domesticated (Smith 1969). As countless anthropological studies and current pet-keeping habits evidence, exotic mammalian, avian and reptilian species are often kept as tame pets, though one could not in any sense describe these creatures as being domesticated or amenable to domestication. Modern endeavours to extend the range of animal domesticates, such as the experimental herding of various species of African antelope, have also proved unsuccessful (Davis 1987: 126–7). The failure to successfully domesticate other species such as the antelope can be linked to several factors. Clutton-Brock (1987) argues that in order for a species to be domesticated, the following five criteria must be met:

1 The animal species chosen must be useful to human society.
2 A species must be adaptive to any environmental changes that might occur as a result of living within human society.
3 Like humans, a species must be social in nature and its behavioural structure should be based on a dominance hierarchy, which will allow it to accept humans as a leader.
4 A species should be able to breed readily and freely within the restricted territory which humans have determined for them.
5 The species must be easy to tend, control and maintain.

The independence, large inter-individual distance, strong sense of territory and substantial feeding range of antelopes makes them a particularly difficult species to herd. Although potentially useful to human society, the failure of the antelope to meet all of the above criteria renders the species unsuitable for domestication (Davis 1987: 127). Whilst such animals might not feasibly be raised as livestock or fully incorporated into human society, they can still be exploited as a resource by humans as game and their territory has been increasingly determined by humans due to urban development and, more recently, the establishment of protected nature reserves or national parks. One could thus say that rather than being domesticated, such species are 'culturally controlled' (Hecker 1982: 219).[3]

As the above suggests, very few species have behavioural characteristics amenable to domestication; the animal, therefore, plays a crucial role in the domestication process. As Bökönyi (1989) observes, domestication is a symbiotic process requiring at least two partners; it cannot be viewed from the side of one of those partners alone. Domestication, he argues, is 'a special kind of symbiosis in the sense that one of the partners, man, influences the other by isolating, taming, controlling, breeding, and taking animals into new habitats, etc., but the animal itself also plays an essential part in this process' (Bökönyi 1989: 24). Although Bökönyi here refers exclusively to the behavioural characteristics of animals and their potential for domestication, his plea to examine domestication from both sides of the fence can be extended much further. It has recently been suggested that by looking at animal domestication from the animal's point of view – rather than thinking about it purely in terms of how it benefited our own species – some of the intricacies of the domestication process might be unravelled. Rather than looking at domestication purely in terms of the human exploitation and subjugation of species, it has been proposed that we should instead seriously consider the extent to which domesticated animals have profited from their seemingly unholy domestic alliance with humankind. Domestication should thus be regarded as a natural product of evolution, rather than the consequence of human innovation.

This alternative view of domestication has gained significant ground in recent years. David Rindos (1984), for example, an evolutionary theorist, has attempted to explain domestication and the origins of agriculture by highlighting the mechanisms of biological, rather than cultural, change. Although Rindos focuses chiefly on the process of plant domestication, his ideas can be extended to encompass the domestication of animal species. To this end, Stephen Budiansky (1992) has drawn inspiration from Rindos' work and has attempted to shed new light on the animal domestication process. Basing his analysis on a wide variety of recent archaeological and animal behaviour studies, Budiansky endeavours to steer away from conventional analyses of domestication by arguing that domestication was an evolutionary strategy not only for humans, but also for particular species of animal. The crux of this argument revolves around the idea that domestication was the result of the cooperative evolution of species as a mutual strategy for survival. Budiansky advances the idea that the adaptability and sociability of these species provide the most important clue to solving the riddle of domestication. The earliest domesticated species – such as dogs, sheep and cattle – were highly opportunistic and did not restrict themselves to a highly specialised terrain or food source; like archaic humans, they too were not loath to exploit new food sources or venture into new realms (Budiansky 1992: 15). The propensity to adapt was imperative for these species' survival, particularly during the Pleistocene when vast environmental and climatic changes occurred, threatening many species with extinction. It was necessary for species to develop cooperative associations with others in order to ensure their own survival. In the long term, this entailed undergoing specific genetic and behavioural changes that would make cooperation easier.

Neoteny, the retention of juvenile traits into adulthood – a feature of all domesticated animals and humans also – was probably the most important of these adaptations. The curiosity and appearance of young animals, their willingness to freely associate with members of other species and care-soliciting behaviour are characteristics that domesticated animals continue to display during adulthood. Such traits probably made them far more malleable and willing to consort with humans than species that did not experience a perpetual youth (Budiansky 1992: 80). In addition to this, the majority of species that were domesticated shared similar social and behavioural traits with humans. Wild dogs, sheep, cattle and horses, for example, live in groups, which have a social hierarchy similar to humans, with a defined social rank and means of expressing dominance and submission recognisable to other species. Furthermore, ungulate species have a clear disposition to follow a dominant animal around. If a human is accepted as a dominant member of the animal group, then the rest of the herd or flock is instinctively inclined to cooperate with him. Finally, domesticated species have a tendency to groom one another and tend to solicit and tolerate the attentions of others who might scratch their backs or remove parasites (Budiansky 1992: 65–7). For the cat, the only domesticated species which did not naturally live within defined social groups or hierarchies, the close association with humans was simply one of social parasitism, although the species also underwent neotenisation (Budiansky 1992: 98–100). In short, Budiansky contends that it was these traits and social affinities that naturally laid the foundations for the domestication process and made intra-species cooperation possible.

Leaving aside the issue of exactly how and why domestication took place, it is reasonable to conclude that the incorporation of other species into human social organisation through the processes of domestication and selective breeding instigated a crucial and irreversible transformation in humankind's relationship with other creatures. By deliberately manipulating and interfering with the natural selection of other animals, humans gained a degree of control over the destiny of other species. Once tamed and segregated from their wild conspecifics, domesticated species could only reproduce within the bounds of human desire and requirements; even their food supply and organisation of territory were determined by their human keepers (Bökönyi 1969; Clutton-Brock 1987; Hemmer 1990; Ucko and Dimbleby 1969). While 'freedom' was the price which animals had to pay for domestication, it could be argued that other species got a pretty good deal from their tacit covenant with their human 'oppressors': they were fed, sheltered, protected from predators; thus their proliferation and survival as species was ensured. Budiansky in particular lauds the success of this seemingly unholy domestic alliance by pointing out that domesticated animals today flourish, while their wild cousins are on the edge of extinction (Budiansky 1992: 61). Others are more doubtful as to whether thriving numbers can be equated with success, given the loss of both genetic diversity and autonomy which animals have suffered as a consequence of their enfoldment into human society (Clutton-Brock 1994).

Finally, the fact that animal domestication also marks an important cultural turning-point for humankind must not be overlooked. The notion that other living animals could be the objects of human ownership not only altered the equilibrium between humans and other species, but also led to significant changes in relationships between humans themselves as the concept and issues of property emerged. Domestication thus resulted in the increasing differentiation, in terms of both behaviour and power, amongst and within human societies (Goudsblom 1992). This ultimately led to specialisation of labour and the development of complex systems of social stratification based on who owned and controlled agricultural resources and who maintained them as underlings, in servitude or wage slavery. In the following, the effects of animal domestication on human social life will be considered in greater detail. As will the profound and unanticipated consequences which the domestication of animals had for the future physical health and well-being of humankind.

The unforeseen consequences of domestication: new risks and responsibilities

The popular characterisation – as advanced by Childe – of the inception of agriculture as a major cultural 'revolution' for humankind is a rather deceptive one. It would in fact take several generations before those human groups who adopted the agrarian regime would begin to truly reap the benefits of domestication or depend exclusively on meat and milk from domesticated animals as dietary staples. Archaeological findings strongly suggest that hunting and gathering continued in a fairly big way alongside agriculture for many generations. Thus, although certain species had been domesticated, it seems that domesticated animals did not play a particularly great role in sustaining human populations until long after their original domestication (Budiansky 1992: 37–8). The amount of produce acquired through hunting and gathering was marginalised and inevitably diminished as agriculture and livestock husbandry advanced (Goudsblom 1992: 42). Furthermore, as will shortly be discussed, the exploitation of, and eventual dependence on, animal resources were to have unanticipated and far-reaching consequences for humankind. In retrospect, the agricultural revolution was perhaps not such a great step forward for humankind as it was once thought. In fact, at least for the first few thousand years, dependence on agriculture and animal husbandry probably presented a far more precarious existence than the hunting and foraging of the past: agriculture is a much more labour-intensive activity that in addition does not necessarily guarantee a continual supply of food.

The agrarian regime entailed radical changes for all those who adopted it. The chief advantage of agriculture was clearly that food could be produced intensively and would – in principle – supply the nutritional needs of ever-growing populations. The increased control over the natural environment which the domestication of both plants and animals offered eventually led to increases in the amount of food available and consequently to increasing human numbers. In order to feed the growing human population, increasingly more food was required. This led to the clearance of virgin land, thus reducing the range of undomesticated territory in which people could hunt or gather their food. In this way, it has been argued, agriculture became increasingly relied on as the sole means of subsistence, for it led to the eradication of other competing systems of obtaining food (Goudsblom 1989a: 21–2). Thus, once agriculture had taken off, there was no way of reverting to the old manner of subsistence. As Budiansky suggests, instead of being a revolution, the rise of agriculture was a 'slow subversion' that, once initiated, could not be stopped (Budiansky 1992: 113).

However, in comparison to the relatively straightforward existence presented by hunting and gathering, tilling the land and maintaining livestock were hard work. Furthermore, dependence on the agricultural mode of food production greatly increased human health risks. Not only were those involved in agriculture prone to new forms of physical injury – for example, skeletal deformities may have been caused by carrying heavy loads – but they also ran a much greater risk of malnutrition and disease. The agricultural lifestyle unavoidably resulted in nutritional problems and deficiencies, which, in turn, would reduce the individual's capacity to look after crops and livestock. Previously, hunting and gathering had offered a more varied diet from diverse food sources. In stark contrast, agriculture restricted food sources to the highly specific crops or animal flesh/milk available, the constant supply of which was never guaranteed due to the possibility of drought, crop failure, parasitic infestation and infectious disease. The topic of infectious disease will be returned to shortly in greater detail. First, however, the impact of agrarian life on human social life and social relations will be briefly considered.

As the above suggests, the inception of agriculture heralded the dawn of an onerous new era for humankind. The cultivation of crops and livestock husbandry was not only arduous work, but also necessitated an increased level of cooperation between individuals and, consequently, the formation of more rigorous personal regimes. Increased control and manipulation of the natural environment resulted in a greatly increased dependency on it and, more specifically, the means (i.e. agriculture and livestock husbandry) and social arrangements that were employed to control it. As the agrarian mode of production became more and more heavily relied on to provide sustenance for growing human populations, the need to adequately maintain and improve it grew. In order to secure a reliable food supply, people would have had to depend on and cooperate with each another more than ever before. As a result of this increased interdependence, individuals necessarily learnt to better attune their conduct and actions to those of others. The development of a far greater sense of foresight was required in order to coordinate agricultural activities and ensure that food production would not be jeopardised. Failure to cooperate and adequately regulate behaviour could ultimately result in the needless loss of livestock and crop failure, and increase the risk of starvation for the entire community, not just the individual. These new interdependencies thus led to the evolution of what Norbert Elias (1994) described as a *social constraint towards self restraint*. In other words, there was increasing pressure within incipient agrarian societies for individuals to regulate their own behaviour in accordance with the demands and situation of others. Avarice, indolence and negligence, for example, would have had far-reaching consequences for all. With regard to animal husbandry, this self-discipline would have involved learning how to properly herd livestock, to selectively slaughter and breed animals, to provide food, shelter and the protection of livestock from predators, to ensure that captive animals did not escape and that they remained healthy.

There was, however, a far greater differentiation in lifestyles and food-production than has thus far been suggested. Although the hunter-gatherer lifestyle had become greatly marginalised, there was another important and alternative way of life that evolved alongside agriculture which involved neither the drudgery of tilling the land nor the harvesting of crops. While the spread of agrarianism brought the existence of domesticated animals to the attention of the hunting peoples living on the periphery of agricultural society, rather than embracing the agricultural mode of production in its entirety, some of these folk adopted only some elements of it and instead became nomadic herdsmen. Pastoralism was a distinctly new way of life, but one that to a large extent preserved both the independence that hunting had previously offered and a social structure based on kinship. Thus, at the margins of agricultural life – i.e. in grasslands of the European steppes and northern Arabia – an alternative mode of existence evolved; which, like agriculture, depended on the exploitation of domesticated animals. In this way, two distinct forms of human social life came to coexist in the Middle East. It is likely that there was a large degree of interaction between the early agriculturalists and pastoralists. Herdsmen, for example, probably brought their flocks to graze on the stubble left after grain had been harvested. Moreover, they undoubtedly entered into trade relations with one another, for the surpluses that each way of life produced could be consumed by the other. However, as later history would attest, violent conflicts between nomadic pastoralists and farming peasants were probably rife. Once the pastoralists became skilled equestrians, their assaults on agricultural communities became increasingly more effective and they were better able to pillage the fruits of agricultural labour (cf. McNeill 1963: 17–18).

Domestication and the subsequent development of and dependence on livestock husbandry or herding thus resulted in an important change in individual behaviour and the structure of human relationships. As the above discussion suggests, both the agrarianisation process and the emergence of a pastoralist way of life were accompanied by an increasing differentiation in behaviour and power both between individuals and amongst human groups. Within human communities, social hierarchies emerged based on power, property and prestige. As agrarian societies developed, the rank and status of individuals were eventually differentiated according to four main categories: peasants, craftsmen and traders, priests and warriors. The vast majority of people in agrarian societies fell into the first category and resided at the bottom of the social hierarchy: these were the people who tended, rather than owned, the land and animals (Goudsblom 1989c: 79–80). Competition for social dominance increased as individuals began to specialise, leading to the emergence of leaders who were able to exercise greater authority over the rest. It was probably these leaders, particularly priests, who exerted the greatest pressure on others to learn and exercise self-restraint. As Goudsblom (1989b) suggests, priests were largely responsible for mediating farming activities. The knowledge of phenomena outside of human control that might affect livestock and harvests – e.g. seasonal change, floods, drought, parasites – which they purported to possess accorded them a certain degree of power and veneration. Consequently they became both responsible for and relied on to direct and determine when, for instance, seeds should be sown, crops harvested and how animals should be slaughtered

(Goudsblom 1989b: 71–2). However, as agriculture became an entrenched and productive way of life, the role of priests in this respect most likely diminished as farmers themselves learned to manage their own activities and transmitted this knowledge to their kin. Nevertheless, the foundations of organised religion and dependence on priests were established and such religious figures went on to provide spiritual guidance and discipline in other domains.

In addition to changes in individual conduct and power relations within human societies, the transitions from foraging to farming and hunting to herding had significant repercussions for relationships between human groups. The pressure to acquire land increased as human populations continued to grow. The first consequence of this was the marginalisation of those human groups who had not undergone this transition. The intensification of agriculture, however, resulted in increased social pressures and tensions with neighbouring agrarian communities and the nomadic pastoralist groups living on the fringes of agrarian society. In order to survive, settled human groups were compelled to protect their land, livestock and other produce. They were thus required to create organised forms of defence to safeguard their material possessions. The agrarian lifestyle made human settlements far more vulnerable to attack from other groups who might attempt to steal or destroy grain, livestock or other material possessions (Goudsblom 1989c). Undoubtedly, the domestication of horses and the subsequent mastery of the equestrian art would have facilitated raids on neighbouring villages greatly. The ultimate consequence of the competition for and vulnerability of resources was that violence within human societies not only became more common, but that it also took on new and organised forms. With respect to this, greater differentiation occurred within human groups as a specialist class of warriors emerged who would protect their own people's resources and pillage those of neighbouring communities. These warriors, alongside or instead of priests, attained superiority within agrarian societies and became powerful, and sometimes oppressive, leaders. The formation of a professional class of warriors, Goudsblom argues, marked the early stages of the monopolisation of violence within human society. Moreover, it manifests the increasing degree of interdependence between individuals of divergent power, wealth and status. The warriors were the most powerful members of society, yet they were dependent on the peasant farmers to produce food. Conversely, the peasants were dependent on the warrior class to protect their livestock, crops and own lives (Goudsblom 1989c:

84–9). Human lives, however, not only became vulnerable in terms of incursion from outside human forces, the transition to agriculture also exposed them to, perhaps more potent, extra-human forces. The final section of this chapter will deal with the formidable threat to human societies that such non-human forces posed.

The emergence and threat of infectious disease

One of the most significant, though much overlooked, repercussions of animal domestication – and certainly the most relevant for this book – was the advent of infectious disease on an epidemic scale. Like violence, infectious disease was a scourge on early agricultural societies, resulting in great mortality – amongst both animal and human populations – and the disruption of food production. The growing intimacy between humans and other animals and increasing exploitation of animal resources, which ensued as a consequence of domestication, created a set of circumstances under which disease-causing microorganisms could flourish and transfer to, and between, human populations on a scale never before possible.

As the historian William H. McNeill explains, the increasing human manipulation and control of the natural world resulted in the disturbance of ecological balances; much in the same fashion as disease organisms upset the natural biological balance within a host's body (McNeill 1976: 29). To a large extent, our hominid and early human ancestors would have been integrated into the natural ecosystem in which they lived, much the same as any other mammalian species (Burnet and White 1972: 138). As our ancestors evolved, they developed into accomplished hunters and, by doing so, achieved a more or less supreme and unchallenged position in the animal kingdom. Within the African heartland, these formidable early human hunters probably maintained a relatively stable relationship to the natural environment (McNeill 1976: 29). However, once they began to intrude into ecosystems within which they had not evolved, humans began to play real havoc with the delicate balances of nature (Burnet and White 1972: 138). Early humans became very successful in exploiting the environment, creating multitudinous new niches for themselves in places and climates that had hitherto been unsuitable for human habitation. Both the domestication of fire and the use of animal skins and fur as clothing allowed humans to survive in colder climates and hunt animal populations previously untouched by human predation.

Once established in these areas, humans successfully used the natural resources and species found there to their advantage.

Human expansionism and the ever-increasing exploitation of natural resources inevitably resulted in the alteration of pre-existing patterns of plant and animal distribution. As human groups began to adopt a sedentary lifestyle and produce their food through agriculture and livestock husbandry, the ecosystems where humans settled were to be changed irrevocably. In the long run, the human manipulation of plants and animals meant that there were larger numbers of fewer species in areas where human settlements were located. This, in turn, created a happy hunting ground for disease-producing parasites, which took great advantage of the new ecological niches created by people. The increasing densities of human populations offered a new food supply to disease organisms. Furthermore, the livestock kept by human communities and the wild scavengers that settlements attracted acted as ideal reservoirs for the microorganisms that would go on to blight human populations (McNeill 1976: 35–56). Hence, although they had achieved a supreme and more or less unchallenged position in the food chain by becoming highly skilled hunters and later agriculturalists, humans remained at peril from predators of a quite different kind: disease-producing microorganisms. These predators would in fact turn out to be potentially more devastating than any of the ferocious beasts that had already been faced in the gradual ascent of the food chain. It is rather ironic that it was humankind's very evolutionary success and mastery of the natural environment which laid them bare to their new microscopic enemies.

This of course is not to say that prior to sedentism disease never afflicted human beings. As discussed earlier in this chapter, a wide variety of food-borne parasites and pathogens would have caused sickness and death in our pre-agrarian ancestors, in addition to rendering them easier prey for other predators. Further to this, bacterial and viral infections would have almost certainly struck the hunter-gatherers of earlier times. Unsanitary living conditions would undoubtedly have been most favourable for the spread of enteric diseases; numerous individuals sharing cramped living quarters, particularly during winter time, would also have provided the ideal conditions for the spread of respiratory infection (Fiennes 1978: 14). Nevertheless, before the inception of agriculture, the microorganisms that caused epidemic disease would have had little opportunity to flourish for long within human communities or to decimate large populations since there were insufficient human or animal reservoirs to harbour and perpetuate disease.

Humans, and our hominid ancestors, lived in relatively small groups, moving around nomadically in search of food. Consequently, many infections, particularly those that are transmitted by droplets, could not spread between human groups easily. Likewise, given this lifestyle, infection would not have been readily acquired from contact with faeces or other waste. Faeces and other refuse would have been dispersed over a wide area, rather than concentrated in one particular or fixed area. If humans were afflicted by infection, the whole group probably suffered and, in the worst scenario, might even have been wiped out entirely. Nonetheless, only a limited number of individuals would have been affected (Zivanovic 1982: 224). Given the small group size and restricted external contacts, disease would simply have died out before it could become virulent or affect large numbers of people. As Cockburn suggests, 'for each infection and set of circumstances, there is a minimum threshold of host population; if the population falls below this threshold, the infection will die out. As a result, the acuteness of an infection is related to the size of the "herd"; small, isolated populations have chronic infections and large ones have more acute infections' (Cockburn 1963: 66). As humans began to adopt a sedentary lifestyle, the numbers of people living together in single locations increased, culminating in a greater concentration of and proximity to the middens and excreta which might harbour infection. Likewise, as the density of settlements increased, harmful pathogens could spread more easily. For example, droplet infections which originated in a single individual could more easily attack a larger number of people who had come into contact with that person – and subsequently those who came into contact with newly infected individuals – leading to a high rate of death and infirmity (Zivanovic 1982: 224).

As the above discussion illustrates, the relationship between humans and disease is one of socio-ecological dynamics. The changing configurations of humans, animals and microorganisms that resulted from increasing human mastery over the natural world opened a new chapter in disease history. The processes of domestication and agrarianisation, therefore, led not only to fundamental and irrevocable transformations in the relationship between humans and other animals, but also altered the symbiosis between parasites and their hosts radically. As McNeill (1976) has argued, from the dawn of agrarianism onwards, disease and civilisation were to become inseparable. The establishment and advance (or fall) of human civilisations, he contends, inescapably went hand in hand with the advance of disease. While humankind flourished and multiplied so did disease-causing organisms. In short, epidemic infectious disease can only exist in what we commonly call 'civilised' communities; in large, complexly organised and densely populated areas where infection passes freely and unceasingly from individual to individual without necessarily even requiring an intermediate host (McNeill 1976: 54).

Thus, while the enfoldment of other species into human society through domestication created – in the long term – a more stable future for humankind, the new-found intimacy between human and beast also created the ideal conditions for the spread of infectious disease on an epidemic scale (Zivanovic 1982: 245). Furthermore, it is most likely that the animals that were domesticated were already the carriers of chronic infection (McNeill 1976: 58). Again, the problem spawned by domestication was one of socio-ecological dynamics. With disease organisms only being able to survive at high population densities, the vast and gregarious herds in which wild cattle, sheep and horses lived prior to domestication had provided the suitable conditions for chains of infection to persist, transferring from animal to animal and between generations. In this way the biological balances between animals and disease-causing parasites had, over the course of time, become more or less stable. The genetic immunity against the effects of contamination that had been acquired by these animals over many generations meant that infections within wild herds probably only appeared in mild or relatively harmless forms. The symptoms which the wild animals exhibited were likely akin to 'childhood diseases' which, while potentially debilitating, are generally not lethal to the afflicted (McNeill 1976: 58–9). However, once these contaminated animals were brought to live within the realms of human social organisation, the relatively innocuous microorganisms that the animals bore acquired a far more deadly and virulent character for there, within human settlements, were large, vulnerable human populations off which they could feed. With little or no immunity against them, initial contact with new disease organisms would probably have been near-catastrophic for the early domesticators. An ongoing relationship between parasite and host would need to be established over a period of centuries before sufficient immunities were built up. Only then would infection become as endemic to humans as it had been to the original animal carriers of the disease (McNeill 1976; Zivanovic 1982).

McNeill argues that it is likely that 'most and probably all of the distinctive infectious diseases of civilisation transferred to human populations from animal herds' (McNeill 1976: 54). The most common infectious diseases, such as measles, influenza and smallpox, which have afflicted humans throughout the ages, closely resemble diseases which affect domesticated animals. Such human diseases can share a common ancestry with animal ones. Measles, rinderpest and distemper, for example, are all caused by pseudomyxoviruses; these three viruses are very closely related and even share common antigens. As Fiennes (1978: 18–19) explains, people who have suffered from measles tend to have antibodies in their sera which neutralise distemper. Likewise, dogs recovering from distemper display antibodies to measles. Although, if exposed to the measles virus, dogs will only produce a minute quantity of antibody to distemper they will, nonetheless, resist the distemper if exposed to it. Similarly, sera taken from cattle immune to rinderpest can neutralise both measles and distemper. Moreover, humans suffering from measles can develop antibodies against rinderpest, and the rinderpest virus has immunising properties against canine distemper. Fiennes suggests that, due to its great virulence in cattle and the lack of apparent wildlife reservoirs for the disease, rinderpest is a relatively recent disease. Measles and rinderpest, he argues, have evolved in humans and cattle respectively as mutations of the distemper virus originally acquired from dogs, which themselves inherited the disease from their lupine ancestors (Fiennes 1978: 19). Similarly, there are clear connections between smallpox in humans and cowpox in cattle, and influenza in both humans and swine (McNeill 1976: 54–5).

Besides these diseases, there exists a large and important group of diseases, known as the zoonoses, which affect humans and the domesticated animals with which they share their lives. A zoonosis is a disease or infection that can naturally be transmitted between vertebrate animals and humans (Schwabe 1984a; Steele 1977; Fiennes 1978). Tuberculosis, as discussed earlier, is one such disease. Humans first probably acquired the tuberculosis parasite through a close association with cattle. While closely related, the bovine and human tuberculosis bacilli are distinct and cause different clinical manifestations in each species (Manchester 1984: 162–3). The bovine variant is, however, also capable of producing the disease in humans. Moreover, humans can act as a reservoir for *Mycobacterium tuberculosis bovis* and reintroduce it into livestock populations that are tuberculosis-free (Brothwell 1991: 18). Other zoonoses of known ancient origin are, for example, rabies and anthrax. Humankind's close association with dogs and meat-eating habits have provided the respective conditions under which these diseases can be transferred to human subjects. The increasing exploitation of animal domesticates also created new opportunities for the transmission of infection from animals to humans. Once humans began to exploit ruminants for their milk, a new and effective path for the transfer of zoonotic disease to humans was established through the consumption of dairy produce (Brothwell 1991: 20). With regard to the relationship between animal and human disease, McNeill proposes the maxim that 'the sharing of infection increases with the degree of intimacy that prevails between man and beast' (McNeill 1976: 55). The greater the interdependence and residential proximity of humans and other animals, the greater the potential for disease to affect human–herd health.

The relationship between the human–animal interdependence and vulnerability to disease is a theme that will be constantly returned to, both explicitly and implicitly, throughout this book. In the chapters that follow, I shall continue to explore the nature of humankind's increasing dependency on other animals and the consequences thereof in terms of health and disease. It will be argued that once infectious disease took hold of human communities, became part of everyday life and became associated with the conditions of, particularly food, animals, there arose a clear need to deal effectively with the manifestations of it. Sick animals threatened human food supplies. Conversely, sick humans were unable to harvest and maintain them adequately. In this way, both veterinary and human medicine gained their *raison d'être* (Wilkinson 1992: 2). The domestication of animals thus gave rise to the emergence of a veterinary regime. In the following chapter, I will look more closely at the very first phase of this process, examining how the veterinary regime was improved and increasingly intensified as human dependency on other animals continued to grow and grow.

3

ANIMALS, DISEASE AND HUMAN SOCIAL LIFE

From ancient times to the early modern period

Increasing exploitation and dependence

As the agricultural way of life evolved and spread throughout the ancient Middle East and eventually into Europe also, the hunter-gatherer lifestyle became increasingly marginalised and was supplanted by crop cultivation and livestock husbandry. The human exploitation of animal resources continued to intensify further as the early agriculturalists discovered that the large animals that they had domesticated could be far more than just walking larders. Indeed, they found that these animals could help them cultivate the plant foods on which they depended and would save them a great deal of backbreaking work in the process. Attaching ploughs to the horns of cattle, particularly oxen, proved to be a significant technological advance, for it allowed fields to be ploughed and kept fallow with far greater ease. The first evidence of traction ploughs dates back to around 3000 BC, though it is likely such ploughs probably were in use before this date. Sumerian pictograms and cylinder seals dating from the end of the fourth millennium BC first record the use of cattle power. Palaeopathological analysis of cattle bones has also suggested stress-induced conditions that might have been associated with the use of animals for traction (Sherratt 1981, 1983).

The harnessing of animal power established a far closer relationship between animal husbandry and crop cultivation, leading to the predominance of mixed farming. Moreover, animal-drawn ploughs facilitated the further expansion of agriculture, for they made the exploitation of difficult soil types possible for migratory farmers. Eventually, other species, such as asses, donkeys and later camels, were also harnessed and used as beasts of burden. Such pack animals could be used to transport agricultural produce over considerable distances and made trading with neighbouring or distant communities much easier. Smaller domesticated species, i.e. dogs, sheep and goats, might also have been used by early agriculturalists to pull and carry small loads (Davis 1987: 162). Later, a far swifter beast, the horse, would come to be harnessed, ridden or employed to pull vehicles such as carts and war chariots. Though for many centuries, as will shortly be illustrated, this species was more the vehicle of warriors than farmers.

Apart from muscle power, the early agriculturalists also came to realise that their animals could be exploited for far more than just flesh, hide, blood, gut and bones. Over time, there was a gradual shift of emphasis within human societies from keeping animals to procure meat and the other by-products of slaughter, to obtaining useful products from the animal throughout the course of its entire life. Animals were thus increasingly exploited for their secondary products: namely milk, fibres and dung. The advent of dairying was a particularly important advance for early agricultural communities. Livestock, i.e. sheep, goats, cattle and also later horses, could be more efficiently exploited to provide protein and energy. Males not required for breeding could still be slaughtered for meat, as could old unproductive females. Dairying was also a far more efficient form of exploitation, for it could yield between four and five times the amount of protein and energy for the amount of fodder consumed as would exploitation for meat production (Sherratt 1981: 284). Nutritionally speaking, milk would not only have provided the early agriculturalists with a good source of fat, protein and sugar, but also with calcium and vitamin D. Milk also had other advantages over meat; not only was it transportable, but it could also be transformed into produce, such as yoghurt, butter and cheese, which were both storable and tradable (Davis 1987: 155–6). The practice of drinking cow's milk, particularly by human babies, Schwabe (1984b) suggests, created an intense bond between humans and other animals; by seeking the milk of another species to nourish their young, humans were effectively using cattle as wet-nurses. The consumption of milk and dairy produce, however, also had its downside. By drinking milk, a new route of transmission for disease-causing pathogens was created (Brothwell 1991: 20).

A second important secondary product of live animals is natural fibre. It is unnecessary to slaughter sheep and goats in order to obtain their wool, instead it can be brushed or sheared away from the animal's body. Selective breeding of sheep gradually transformed ovine coats from bristly hairs to soft fleeces. Goats were probably less frequently used for wool production and their coats have consequently been altered little by selective breeding with an eye to the production of textiles. Ordinary goat hair can be woven into a coarse cloth, whereas the underwool of a moulting goat can be used to produce cashmere (Davis 1987: 156). The emergence of wool use is coincidental to the inception of urban development in Mesopotamia. Woollen textiles would have been merchantable goods and were probably used to obtain other produce or metals unavailable locally. However, like milk, handling animals' fleeces and wool may have been deleterious to human health. Serious infectious diseases, such as anthrax, were likely transmitted through this close association with sheep and goats. Finally, the third important by-product of living animals that the early agriculturalists began to utilise was their dung. Animal excreta can be used very effectively as manure to enrich the quality and fertility of the land. The importance of dung for crop cultivation illustrates the great interdependence of agricultural practices. Grain production was contingent on the exploitation of this secondary product of livestock husbandry. In ancient times, dung and droppings may also have been used, as they were in later societies, for medicinal purposes. By handling, and possibly even ingesting, animal faeces, people would also have exposed themselves to a variety of parasites that may have caused infection and disease.

It is evident that as the exploitation of domesticated animals as a resource increased, so did human dependency on them and vulnerability to disease also. Livestock, as Jared Diamond (1997: 195–214) puts it, increasingly proved to be a 'lethal gift' to humankind. This chapter will continue to explore the increasing diversification and intensification of animal use from antiquity up until the early modern period. Moreover, it will look at the ever-increasing importance of domesticated species to human societies and the repercussions thereof. In this regard, I shall elaborate on the theme of dependency and disease that was introduced in the previous chapter, by further examining the devastating effects of animal disease on agricultural society. In particular, the impact of epizootics on the agricultural economy will be the focus of discussion. As a corollary to this, the final part of this chapter will be devoted to an exploration of early animal medicine and the evolution of an incipient veterinary regime.

Animals in ancient societies

The increased manipulation and growing importance of living animals to human society led to an increasingly high value being placed on livestock. Animals signified wealth. Furthermore, the importance of animals to human society increasingly came to be reflected in the spiritual beliefs and religious teachings of ancient societies. The earliest known cultures appear to have been highly zoocentric in nature. Sheep were probably the first agricultural animals to be domesticated and it is likely that early pastoralist culture and religion revolved around this species. Ancient Judaic culture, for example, appears to have been centred around this species. The Old Testament in particular is laden with ovine imagery. Allegorical tales of God as a shepherd and people as his flock abound in this holy book; the shepherd can be perceived as a paragon of virtue and humanity to which the Jewish people should aspire (Schwabe 1994: 49). Early Jewish tribes were undoubtedly not the only peoples in the Middle East who were dependent on sheep and built their culture and religion around them. The Bible, with its stories of the trials and tribulations of the Jewish people, preserves the only tangible written record of such a sheep culture. Interestingly, as Schwabe (1978: 11) observes, these 'sheep people' were eventually forced to struggle to preserve their existence as they came into confrontation with other settled groups, such as the Egyptians, Canaanite-Phoenicians and Babylonians, among whom they lived. Unlike the Jews, these ancient peoples possessed the trappings of 'civilised' life and centred their spiritual life around a quite different species: cattle.

Cattle herding was an important preoccupation for the ancient peoples of Mesopotamia and Egypt. Their dependence on cattle for muscle power, secondary produce and meat endowed these animals with an important status. Cattle signified wealth, power and fertility, and accordingly they were revered, anthropomorphised and transformed into the objects of worship. These animals are predominant in the pantheons of Sumerian and other early Mesopotamian peoples, such as the Chaldeans, Assyrians, Hittites and Akkadians. Bull gods and cow goddesses appear to have played a central role in ancient Mesopotamian religion. It has even been suggested that cattle houses, originally constructed from reed, provided the model on which more permanent and elaborate temple architecture was based (Schwabe 1978, 1994). These temples were quite literally considered the homes of the gods and much of the society's economic life centred around them, until more militarised and secular forms of government arose (McNeill 1963: 34–6). Bovine imagery also pervaded ancient Egyptian religious thought and art, leading entire cults to be built up around cattle. Schwabe (1994) has suggested that such bovine imagery derived originally from the Egyptians' anatomical, physiological, behavioural and social observations of cattle. He has argued that the Egyptian kings – who were seen as gods incarnate in human form – wished to emulate the mighty and libidinous bulls that dominated cattle herds. By analogy, the pharaoh ruled over his human herd with bovine vigour. The ancient Egyptians perceived the bull's horns and penis as the source of the animal's great power. Schwabe contends that much of the symbolism relating to the pharaoh's might derives anatomically from the bull's horns or reproductive organs (Schwabe 1994:43–4).[1]

Further to their spiritual significance, an interesting theory has been forwarded which postulates that the accumulation of cattle wealth was a critical factor in the formation of the dynastic Egyptian state. Lobban (1989) has suggested that cattle provided the capital that permitted the accumulation of wealth, social differentiation and urbanisation in ancient Egypt, not to mention the financing of monumental construction. This cattle wealth, he argues, was largely acquired through military force, from violently raiding their southerly Nubian neighbours. Lobban contends that the success and frequency of these raids created an urgent need to increase agricultural production; not to meet human food needs, but instead to provide for those of animals. Animals, as he observes, are far greater consumers of agricultural produce than humans. Cattle in particular require enormous quantities of fodder to remain healthy and productive. Although additional agricultural produce was certainly necessary to feed the slaves also captured during the cattle raids and the military force which made them captive, this was minimal in comparison to the amount of food necessary to maintain the rapidly growing and increasingly valuable livestock population. Lobban thus contends that the intensification of agricultural production in the Nile delta developed in order to provide fodder for cattle; only later did crop cultivation grow in importance as a human food supply. In short, he has argued that the development of organised and frequent military assaults on neighbours, combined with the resulting huge increase in livestock numbers, precipitated the process of state formation in ancient Egypt (Lobban 1989: 197–9).

Cattle thus played an important role within the ancient societies of the Middle East. However, as the diffusion of civilisation continued into southern Europe, leading to the emergence of the Greek and Roman civilisations, cattle became relegated to a lower position in society; used almost exclusively for agriculture, traction and food. It was to be another, later domesticate, the horse, that came to usurp the holy cow and sacred bull. Though unlike cattle, the horse did not receive the same kind of spiritual attention. Instead, this species took on an important military and mercantile function, allowing its masters to travel increasingly long distances to trade with and vanquish – and often enslave – other less powerful and mobile peoples. In early Greek times, the role of horseback soldiers was crucial in battle for they could move swiftly and were able to thwart the efforts of their rivals' foot-soldiers. But only the wealthy had the means to become cavalrymen, because horses were necessarily grain-fed throughout most of the year due to a dearth of natural grass in Greece. Thus as the importance of the cavalry grew, the aristocratic landowners increased their leverage in public affairs (McNeill 1963: 196). By the late seventh and sixth century BC, however, the cavalry was supplanted as the ultimate force on the battlefield. Cavalrymen were replaced by 'hoplites', heavily weaponed and armoured infantrymen, who rhythmically moved in a massed military formation known as a phalanx. Even men on horseback found it difficult to break up this disciplined human formation (McNeill 1963: 198).[2] Horses and chariots were thus generally only used to transport the hoplites to the battleground, and were left with attendants away from the front line during fighting (Clutton-Brock 1992: 108). The Roman army also required a reliable supply of mounts – along with men with the appropriate equestrian skills to ride them – for its military campaigns, which meant that horse breeding became an important business within Roman society. Yet although the cavalry was crucial to Roman warfare, only a small proportion of each legion were actually cavalrymen (Clutton-Brock 1992: 115). Horses – and their riders – were specially trained for military purposes and were fitted with various kinds of armour that had been especially designed to protect them from injury during battle and probably to aid the intimidation of peasants also (Azzaroli 1985; Hyland 1990; Dixon and Southern 1992).

The horse also became the pride and joy of the rich and free in both these ancient societies, being widely used for their sporting pleasure. This marks a significant historical development in the use of horses. As Azzaroli observes, the Greeks appear to have been the first people to develop their equestrian skill simply for the sake of the 'sheer pleasure of riding on horseback' (Azzaroli 1985: 52). The ancient Greeks excelled in the art of sporting equitation and chariot racing. In addition to their use in games and races, they employed their horses for travel, hunting wild game and also for ceremonial purposes such as parades and religious processions (Anderson 1961). Likewise, horses were ridden within Roman society for pleasure, hunting game, travel, ceremony and racing in the circuses. Other equids, such as asses and mules, also carried riders and were employed as pack animals, or to haul carts, for land transport and postal services. Donkeys were used to work reaping machines and, in later times, water mills also (Toynbee 1973: 15). Ass's milk was, of course, a renowned ingredient of Roman beauty baths (Barclay 1980: 57).

Food-producing animals were a valuable commodity in both ancient Greece and Rome. The mountainous Greek landscape particularly lent itself to the herding of sheep and goats. Shepherds, who often had to move their flocks across considerable distances from summer to winter pastures, supplied towns and cities with meat and cheese (Ryder 1983). The right of freemen to pasture sheep was determined by the polis, and fines were issued for overgrazing. Cooperation between city states was in some cases necessary due to the distances shepherds had to travel and the land available for pasture. The grazing of sheep was therefore at times a political issue that could cause friction between city states. Sheep were also important for textile manufacturing. The wool that they produced was sorted, spun and woven into cloth, which sometimes also underwent a dyeing process before being transformed into clothing (Ryder 1983: 156). Shepherds would also be accompanied by dogs for protection against predators. In addition to these species, pigs and cattle were kept by the ancient Greeks as livestock. Oxen were used to plough the land, and it has even been suggested that teams of yoked oxen were employed to haul the large stones that they used to construct their temples (Dunlop and Williams 1996: 138).

Oxen were also perhaps the most valuable domesticated species to the Romans for they depended heavily on these animals to plough their fields. Cattle were thus selectively bred to produce the bovine characteristics most suitable for pulling ploughs and other heavy draught purposes. In this regard, it was recommended that cattle under two years old should not be castrated; late castration would lead to greater growth which would be advantageous in animals used for draught. Interestingly, although cattle were milked, there does not appear to have been great concern for milk production. Veal production, however, was a source of the Roman cattle breeders' income, far more so than beef which is rarely mentioned in documents relating to the Roman diet. Steers that were not trained to be yoked were sold for sacrifice (Walker 1973: 323–5). Sheep husbandry was also vital to the Roman agricultural economy. Milk and wool were then the main yield of sheep, their meat was held to be of secondary importance. To a large extent it was the setting of a farm that determined whether or not lambs were sent to slaughter. If they grazed in distant pastures, it was simply not profitable enough to transport these animals to towns for slaughter. Lambs were at times offered for sacrifice, providing another potential market for sheep breeders (Ryder 1983). Again, dogs were employed to protect and manage flocks of sheep, as well as being used as guard or watch dogs, for hunting and being kept as pets within Roman society.

In addition to cattle, sheep and dogs, the Romans kept goats and pigs. Pigs were sometimes fattened on the surplus of wheat bran produced by milling white bread. Boars were typically castrated at approximately six months of age (Walker 1973: 329–30). Pig meat was generally preserved by either smoking or salting. While pig products were apparently popular with Romans of all social classes, they were an essential constituent of the diet of the urban poor. Pigs breed quickly and eat cheaply on human food debris, so even the poorest farmers could probably afford to keep one or more of them (Barker 1985: 34–5). However, the popularity and profusion of pig produce in the Roman diet – along with the butchering and consumption of diseased animals – put Romans, of all classes, at risk of serious infectious diseases such as anthrax (Walker 1973: 330). The Romans' idiosyncratic partiality to eating the humble dormouse as a delicacy led to these rodents being deliberately fattened on chestnuts, acorns or walnuts in special 'farms' (Hooper and Ash 1934).

Increasing exploitation: from the Middle Ages to the early modern period

The Middle Ages bore witness to a gradual, but significant change in attitudes towards animals and a reconsideration of the human relationship to them.[3] The expansion of Christianity throughout Europe during the early Middle Ages, for example, led to the widespread repudiation of existing pagan beliefs in the close proximity of humans and animals. Within Christian thought, humans and animals were perceived as being qualitatively different from each other; animals could be principally distinguished from humans by their lack of reason and their want of an immortal soul (Salisbury 1994: 4–6). Yet while philosophical ideas about animals began to change, the exploitation of animals continued in much the same fashion as it had done for several thousand years. Draught animals, particularly oxen, were crucial to the mediaeval farmers who relied on them to plough their fields and to pull heavy loads (Langdon 1986). The critical importance of cattle to mediaeval society was clearly reflected in the legal codes of the time, which sought to protect the potential labour of animals from being compromised. Visigothic law (476–654), for example, stipulated that any person who mutilated someone else's animal would be ordered to replace it with one of equal value. Overworking an animal borrowed for the purposes of draught also met with a penalty, for the owner would have to be compensated for the reduction in capacity of his own beast. Similar penalties and laws for compensation were also reflected in the legal codes of the Alamans and the Franks (Salisbury 1994: 19). Although care was advised in order to exploit animal labour to the full, oxen were yoked and worked to their limits, usually for a period of about four years, until they were exhausted or no longer physically capable of fulfilling their tasks, after which time they were fed up and sold for slaughter and profit (Salisbury 1994: 20–1).

The early Middle Ages also bore witness to the increasing diversification of horse use within European society. Although horses retained and even grew in military importance and continued to be employed for hunting and sporting purposes by the nobility, during the mediaeval period the equine species increasingly began to be employed as working animals alongside oxen. Horses were thus employed to pull carts and used for transportation. Moreover, they began to be used instead of oxen for ploughing the land. Yet while horses could work much faster and longer than oxen, they were in fact far more expensive to maintain (Langdon 1986). In late-twelfth-century England, mixed teams of horses and oxen were sometimes employed to plough the land, though – apart from north-eastern France where horses replaced oxen and Spain, where mules did the job – oxen continued to maintain their role as the principal animal used for ploughing. Nonetheless, the versatility and stamina of horses presented a particularly attractive proposition to smallholders who could exploit them not only for ploughing or harrowing the land, but also for riding and pulling carts. Unlike cattle, however, they were costly to maintain and did not fetch as good a price as oxen for their flesh and hide when they reached the end of their working lives (Salisbury 1994: 21–2). These draught animals were of supreme importance to the development of European society and agriculture. As Keith Thomas has noted, 'the civilisation of medieval Europe would have been inconceivable without the ox and the horse. Indeed', he writes, 'it has been estimated that the use of animals for draught and burden gave the fifteenth-century European a motor power five times that of his Chinese counterpart' (Thomas 1983: 25).

Next to muscle power, animal hide was also of great importance for the manufacture of shoes, clothing, furnishings and other goods. During the mediaeval period, animals were increasingly exploited for the production of parchment. The best quality parchment, known as vellum, was generally obtained from calves that had been slaughtered while they were still being milk fed. However, the finest quality vellum used to make valuable books such as the Bible came from the skin of foetal calves. Joyce Salisbury (1994) offers the example of the fifteenth-century Gutenberg Bible to illustrate the sheer amount of calfskin necessary to produce such a holy book; she estimates that 'one copy of the Bible required 170 calfskins, so the initial 35 vellum copies required the skins of nearly 6000 calves' (Salisbury 1994: 23). In addition to hide, the natural fibres of living animals were also a valuable commodity to mediaeval society. Sheep wool was in fact to be an important factor in the development of commercialism within European society. Throughout the late Middle Ages, wool provided an increasingly good income and greatly supplanted the other uses of sheep for the production of milk, meat and manure. The wool trade was particularly important in Britain where wool was of good quality and made great profits, for example, from exportation overseas to Flanders where a cloth industry began to flourish from the twelfth century onwards (Salisbury 1994: 26). To meet wool demands, flocks were also fairly extensive; by 1532 they had become so large that the English authorities took measures to restrict flocks to 2,000 sheep. The British wool trade continued to be of great importance into the early modern period and even went on to shape the nation's later colonial activities in Australia and New Zealand. The size of Britain's sheep population also reflects this: in 1741, there were 16.5 million sheep; in 1774, this had increased to 25.5 million and by 1871, there were some 34,532,000 sheep living in the British Isles (Reid 1871: 20).[4]

The exploitation of animals continued to intensify after the Middle Ages. In Britain, this development was typified by the growth of the wool trade. Across the waters of the North Sea in the Netherlands, farmers increasingly came to depend on livestock for their livelihoods as grain production, particularly in coastal areas, became infeasible due to changing soil conditions. From the fourteenth century onwards, livestock keeping and breeding therefore grew in importance, particularly with regard to milk production, leading to the development of a flourishing trade in butter and cheese (Davids 1989: 12–13). By the early sixteenth century, Europe had also acquired a new domesticated species that could be exploited for food: the turkey (Davis 1987: 194). This bird had been imported from the New World that had been 'discovered' following the Columbian voyage of 1492. The conquest of the Americas led not only to the dispersion of European civilisation, but also to the dispersion of animals, plants and disease-causing organisms across the great ocean (Crosby 1994). Alongside their human counterparts, European livestock species and horses came to colonise the American continent. The Spanish conquistadors also saw the Americas as providing a new solution to the stock-raising crisis back home. By the sixteenth century, the Iberian peninsula had become overgrazed and attempts to make room for new pastures on which cattle could graze only led to deforestation. The ever-growing demand for beef and hide put great pressure on Spanish soil, leading to substantial desertification. An opportunity was seized to transfer cattle production to the New World; the cattle imported from the home country also went on to flourish in their new environment (Rifkin 1992: 45).

In the centuries that followed, increasing human food demands – as subsequent chapters will go on to illustrate – led to an inevitable need to intensify livestock production. Since ancient times, animal breeders had tried to selectively breed and refine livestock animals in order to obtain better quality wool, higher milk yields and greater muscle power. The selective breeding of horses had also led to the production of larger horses for mediaeval warfare, eventually leading to the rise of huge varieties of draught animals such as the Shire (Langdon 1986: 17–19). By the seventeenth century, the average size of cattle, sheep, pigs and domestic fowl had greatly increased; meat, in particular, was in ever-greater demand (Davis 1987: 188). It was, however, only to be during the eighteenth century that the improvement of livestock truly became an end in itself. The most renowned pioneer of livestock breeding was Robert Bakewell. Bakewell was the first animal breeder to demonstrate how new breeds of cattle could be produced through the practice of inbreeding and selection. In recognising the increased demand for high-quality beef and tallow – a fat widely used for lighting – Bakewell set out to deliberately select stock that had a propensity for fattening and which matured quickly. His emphasis was on increasing the animal's economic performance and productivity, rather than on its appearance, which was the chief goal of contemporary breeders (Dunlop and Williams 1996: 354–5). Indeed, Bakewell's methods received a great deal of criticism from his contemporaries. Having, for example, produced a breed of sheep – the New (or Dishley) Leicester – which would yield larger quantities of meat, he sacrificed other traits such as wool quality that were viewed by others as desirable and aesthetically pleasing. This 'disposition to produce fat on the most profitable parts', as one critic put it, went against the very notion of animal aestheticism (Thomas 1983: 285–6). Bakewell, however, was to set a trend for the future of livestock breeding and many – some taught by him – followed in his footsteps and went on to produce cattle with a higher milk yield and pigs that fattened more quickly.

Alongside these new breeding practices came also the importation and development of foreign breeds that were known for the quality and quantity of their produce. For instance, Spanish Merino sheep, prized for the quality of their wool, were imported into France during the mid-eighteenth century, partially in order that the French could produce their own wool supply and would no longer be dependent on their Spanish neighbours to furnish them with the raw materials to produce quality cloth. Later Merinos were also imported to Britain and eventually ended up being exported to distant colonies (Ryder 1983: 427; Dunlop and Williams 1996: 356–61). Such sheep were later to become the economic mainstay of Australia and New Zealand, the latter country becoming a leading producer of sheep meat and the former a major world supplier of quality wool (Ryder 1983: 608–41). Imports from Asia also bore witness to changes in another species: the pig. Chinese pigs were cross-bred with the lean and slow-growing European breeds to produce animals that had a propensity to fatten. By the mid-nineteenth century, however, the consumer preference had changed from fat pork to leaner meat, requiring the development of an altogether different kind of porker that would produce the appropriate flesh in the kind of quantities that the consumer increasingly demanded (Wiseman 1986: 77–85). The importation of stock, however, brought with it increased opportunities for the transmission and spread of infectious disease. In the following section, I shall consider the impact that animal disease had on agricultural society from antiquity up until the mid-eighteenth century.

Animal disease in agrarian society

The increasing exploitation of animals led not only to an increasing dependency on them, but also to an increased vulnerability to them. From antiquity onwards, animal disease was to have a devastating effect on agricultural communities. In some respects, it is difficult to gauge the precise impact or nature of the disease that afflicted the earliest agrarian societies. The palaeopathological analysis of bones may sometimes detect evidence of ancient disease; clear signs of tuberculosis infection, for example, have been found in the vertebrae of skeletons over 4,000 years old (Zivanovic 1982: 226–9). Written records may also provide some clues, but they are often vague with regard to the aetiology of disease and the extent to which it may have affected the animal or human population. Furthermore, the diseases that we recognise today were not always clearly differentiated from other conditions. Brucellosis is one such example. Until the nineteenth century, this important zoonotic disease was indistinguishable from malaria and a number of other infections (Brothwell 1991: 21). It is quite probable that brucellosis was the cause of spontaneous abortion in livestock for many centuries, but the most concrete scientific evidence of infection dates back only to the early fifteenth century AD. The microbial agents that cause such disease could also not be identified until very recently, because their proteins generally did not survive. Developments in molecular biology have now provided the means with which their DNA can be detected (Houwers 1994: 27).

It is also possible to speculate on the presence of infectious diseases on the basis of the kind of environmental and demographic conditions that existed in the past. In ancient Mesopotamia and Egypt, for example, the density and proximity of human and animal populations in both the Tigris–Euphrates and Nile river valleys provided the appropriate conditions under which infectious diseases could be spread. Irrigation farming in the warm Middle Eastern climate created an ideal moist environment where parasites could be transferred from host to host (McNeill 1976: 47–8). Schistosomes –

parasitic blood flukes, which infect both livestock and humans – were probably present in the shallow water-irrigated environments of ancient Mesopotamia, as they were in ancient Egypt also. Schistosomiasis, in either humans or animals, would have impeded agricultural production; resulting in disease in farmers and irrigation labourers and possibly even causing the death of sheep and cattle. It is certain that the ancient Egyptians suffered from this condition, because examinations of mummified human tissues have revealed the presence of schistosomal infestations (Adamson 1976: 176–8). Contamination with this blood fluke would have been debilitating for those working in the fields and irrigation channels, reducing their capacity to resist military attack and economic exploitation by others (McNeill 1976: 49).[5] Further to this, the intimate relationship between cattle and humans was doubtless also the source of bacterial infection and disease in ancient Egypt. For example, the trade and herding of cattle would have encouraged the spread of bovine tuberculosis amongst herds, resulting in mortality and loss of production. Moreover, milk supplied from infected cattle may have resulted in the transfer of this bacterial disease to humans. Conclusive evidence of tuberculosis infection has been found in a human mummy dating from the XXIst Dynasty (1070–946 BC) (Manchester 1984: 163–4).

As the previous chapter outlined, the consumption of contaminated animal flesh is a primary cause of human illness. A prime source of animal protein in early Egypt was pig flesh. Human–porcine relations in ancient Egypt were, however, at best ambivalent. In pre-dynastic times, pigs thrived along the marshy banks of the Nile and were a standard foodstuff. The omnivorous pig gives a high energy yield in its fat and flesh, making it an ideal source of animal protein. Yet, within ancient Egypt, a taboo against eating it gradually evolved. The prohibition on eating pig meat has generally been associated with notions of hygiene and infection. McNeill (1976: 50), for example, suggests that the Jewish prohibition of eating pork probably resulted from an 'intuitive horror' of the hogs' scavenging habits – i.e. eating human faeces. Alternative explanations of the prohibition on pork, however, suggest that it may not actually have had anything to do with hygiene at all. Lobban (1994), for example, has argued that the pig taboo in ancient Egypt is closely linked to the process of state formation. As the ecology of the Nile delta was transformed by irrigation to make way for the production of cattle fodder, the species' habitat was destroyed and the pig gradually became marginalised as a less socially desirable food (Lobban 1994: 72). Moreover, as Harris (1977) has asserted, the omnivorous pig was in direct competition with humans for valuable food resources, and was simply too expensive to rear for food. Pigs also did not serve any useful purpose other than as meat producers: the species cannot be milked, ridden, herd other animals, pull ploughs, carry loads or catch rodents. By prohibiting pig rearing, people were encouraged to produce less expensive sources of animal protein and to cultivate crops (Harris 1977: 196–9). Whatever the reasons for the pig taboo, it is certain that there are a variety of diseases that are associated with humans and pigs that were present in antiquity. Trichinosis, a nematode infection, is commonly cited as the reason for the pig taboo. However, *Trichinella spiralis* can affect other livestock species and infection is generally not fatal (Lobban 1994; Meyer 1992). Still, even if it was not the reason for it, the prohibition on pork would have prevented this and other helminthic, bacterial, viral and fungal infections from being transferred from pigs to people (Adamson 1989).

Parasitic and bacterial infections, either affecting animals or transferred from animals to humans, were doubtless a bane on the lives of the ancients. While not necessarily fatal, they could be debilitating and reduce the individual's (human or animal) productive capacity. Epidemic disease, however, would have had more consequential effects on ancient Egyptian society than infections such as trichinosis or schistosomiasis. When pestilence struck the animal population, the results were probably devastating. Even if the infections that afflicted domesticated animals were not zoonotic, they would still have had potentially serious consequences for their human keepers. The hindrance of agricultural production through livestock disease would have resulted in serious economic losses. Cattle diseases, for instance, may have resulted in high mortality amongst animals indispensable for ploughing the fields and producing foodstuffs. Animal disease would thus have resulted in hardship for the peasant agriculturalists, possibly leading to malnutrition or starvation and the reduction of human resistance to other infections (cf. Wilkinson 1992). Little is known about the exact nature of the pestilence that struck the ancient Egyptians. However, in a rather creative epidemiological interpretation of the biblical story of the ten plagues of Egypt, Blaisdell (1994) has suggested that at least seven of these plagues were actually interrelated phenomena involved in an outbreak of anthrax. As one of the oldest known zoonotic diseases, it is quite likely that the ancient

Egyptians and their livestock would have been struck by this terrible disease.

The ancient civilisations of Greece and Rome were also put to the test by the coming of animal plagues. In classical Greek poetry, detailed references can be found to the effects of mythical or real plagues on humans and animals. Homer, for example, chronicled the horrors of an outbreak of plague in 1183 BC in the *Iliad*, assigning responsibility for the catastrophe to the god Apollo – the overseer of flocks and herds within the Greek pantheon – who had 'showered his arrows among them [the people] when displeased, and slew men and beast alike by his vengeful but unseen darts' (quoted in Fleming 1871: xx). An anachronistic interpretation of this story would likely see these darts as a metaphor for the invisible organisms that caused the plague. Homer also outlined the hygienic measures that were taken following this plague. He wrote that in order to cleanse and purify 'filth and obnoxious matter' were thrown into the sea (Fleming 1871: 8). It is possible that such filth simply offended people's sensibilities, although the evolution of a more sophisticated medicine may well have encouraged the improvement of sanitary measures. Whatever the case, it is certain that both epidemic and epizootic disease at times raged throughout Greek cities and the countryside, affecting both humans and livestock and often resulting in shortages in agricultural produce, which led to food crises. The close association between famine and disease was also recognised in Greek times, although they were viewed as divine punishments for the people's profanity (Garnsey 1988: 25–6). Infections, such as the one which precipitated the famous plague of Athens (430–429 BC), as described by Thucydides, were likely transferred through foreign trade across the Mediterranean sea (McNeill 1976: 103).

Similarly, the poets who chronicled the agricultural life of Ancient Rome reveal much about the effects of animal disease on Roman society. In the *Georgics*, Virgil provides a clear description of an outbreak of anthrax and its devastating effects on livestock farmers of the time. In the following, one can see how understanding about the need for hygiene was necessary to prevent disease from spreading from animals to humans. Virgil writes:

> And now they died by whole companies, and the corpses
> Rotting with vile decay lay piled in the very sheep folds,
> Till men had learnt to put them in pits, covered with earth.
> The hide was no good, and no man

> Could cleanse the carcase in water or burn it up with fire:
> You could not even shear the fleece, it was so corroded
> With foul pus, or work that rotten wool in the loom:
> But if you were so foolhardy as to wear the hideous garment,
> Inflamed pustules and a noxious-smelling sweat appeared
> All over your limbs: not long then
> Before the fiery curse ate up your tettered frame.
> (quoted in Steele 1977: 1)

In his chronicles, Virgil describes a wide variety of identifiable animal diseases, ranging from anthrax to sheep scab and rabies. Moreover, he recommends several cures for such diseases and attributes the cause of disease to insanitary conditions. The neglect of hygiene and failure to practise good agriculture almost certainly precipitated plague amongst humans and other animals during Roman times. It is in fact believed that pestilence – amongst both human and animal populations – played an important role in the decline of the Roman Empire. Infections were likely carried by merchant ships and pack trains that regularly crossed from one side of Eurasia to the other, and acquired by soldiers during military campaigns far afield. In short, the expansion of the Roman Empire – in which the horse played a highly significant role – also led to the expansion of opportunities for disease-causing organisms. Exposure to new disease organisms had devastating consequences for the Roman people who had little or no immunity built up to them. Outbreaks of serious epidemic disease were responsible for the decay of the Roman population, resulting in exceptionally high mortality rates, particularly in urban areas, which consequently affected the commercial base of Roman society and its cash flow to support military activities (McNeill 1976: 112–16). Natural disasters, such as volcanic eruptions, earthquakes, locust swarms, drought and flood, also often preceded outbreaks of epidemic and epizootic disease, leading at times to food shortages and famine. As Livy, the prominent Roman historian, observed, disease often began in cattle shortly before it affected human populations (Fleming 1871: 17).

The diseases of domesticated animals continued to periodically afflict and decimate both human and animal populations into the Middle Ages. During the fifth and sixth centuries, several epizootics – that are believed by later authors to have been rinderpest – occurred in western Europe following the horseback incursions of barbarian tribes such as the Huns. Likewise, during the ninth century, Charlemagne's warring activities brought epizootics in their wake. Such animal plagues greatly compromised agricultural production, resulting in high mortality amongst livestock and famine (Fleming 1871; Dunlop and Williams 1996). Again, the advent of such animal plagues provides a sharp reminder that the blight of animal disease is not simply restricted to the infections that cross the species' divide. Perhaps more significant than the direct physical effects of zoonotic diseases, outbreaks of infectious disease amongst domesticated animal populations have often created the conditions under which other infections can affect human populations – sometimes to epidemic proportions – for they have lowered human resistance to disease since they have caused great hardship, scarcity and starvation (Wilkinson 1994).

The devastation that follows or accompanies animal disease is exemplified by the events that shook European society to its very foundations during mediaeval times. By the thirteenth century, the rapidly expanding population had put excessive pressure on land and food resources and infectious disease gained a greater foothold due to changes in human populations and the changing interdependencies between humans and other animals. The outbreaks of bubonic plague that gripped late mediaeval European society are illustrative of the risks posed by the intimacy that exists between humans and domesticated animals. The bacillus *Pasteurella pestis* – as it was later identified and labelled during the late nineteenth century – was responsible for the devastating plague that hit Europe during the mid-fourteenth century. The Black Death (1348–50) was essentially a disease of rats; bubonic plague, and the pneumonic plague which accompanied it, radically affected human populations when the rat fleas which spread the disease left their dead or dying rodents to attack human beings in search of new hosts (Wilkinson 1994: 11–12). New patterns of human movement resulting from military expansionism and increasing commerce eventually brought the plague to Europe from the east. Population upheaval and changes allowed the disease to move from areas and rodent populations where it was presumably endemic to new areas previously unaffected (McNeill 1976).

The human population of Europe was extremely vulnerable at this time. During the early fourteenth century, typhus, influenza and smallpox widely afflicted the human communities. In addition, a number of ecological disasters occurring during this period – including volcanic eruptions in Italy, severe winters and extensive flooding of the Rhône which led to crop failures in France – had also devastated the economy and populace of certain regions. These localised disasters, in turn, precipitated more widespread and rampant plagues – such as rinderpest and anthrax – amongst sheep and cattle, leading to great hardship and famine amongst the wider European human population. With such low resistance and lack of immunity against the new bacterium, *Pasteurella pestis* was able to ravage human communities and destabilise European society (Wilkinson 1992: 22–3). At first, the population decimation did not seem to make too much of a difference to the economy. The rapidly expanding peasant population had already put great pressure on available resources from the thirteenth century onwards leading to deforestation and food shortages. However, when the plague struck again during the 1360s and 1370s, population decay and manpower shortages began to have a significant impact on the agricultural economy (McNeill 1976:156–9). With the spectre of plague hanging over late-mediaeval European society, the need to minimise its effects and the risk of infection became evident and measures began to be taken to attempt to contain future outbreaks through quarantine or avoidance of infected individuals.

At first sight, the Black Death may not seem such a good illustration of the impact of the diseases of domesticated animals on human societies. In this instance, the pestilence was spread to humans by black rats and their parasites, rather than directly from domesticated animals. However, the changing configurations of humans and animals at this time provided a magnet for these scavengers who readily took advantage of new ecological niches created largely by human movements. More importantly, the Black Death exemplifies how epidemics affecting human health have followed hot on the heels of animal plagues. Animal disease has repeatedly increased the vulnerability of human populations to disease organisms. For societies dependent on agriculture and animal husbandry, the effects of animal plagues can be devastating: fragile economies can be shattered, people already living at subsistence level may starve and infectious disease can gain a firm grip and decimate already weakened peoples and social structures.

European society continued to endure the devastating effects of murrain throughout the late Middle Ages and into the early modern period.[6] Farming communities remained more or less helpless in the wake of animal plagues and were consequently faced with great losses amongst livestock. When animal disease struck, people were invariably inclined to regard it as divine punishment or to blame witchcraft for their misfortunes. For example, in sixteenth-century England, the death or injury of animals was frequently attributed to the nefarious activities of witches (L'Estrange Ewen 1933; Macfarlane 1970). By the end of the fifteenth century – with the aid of development of the art of printing – public authorities across Europe began to produce and distribute broadsheets to inform people of the diseases common to cattle and horses (Wilkinson 1992: 24). The agricultural writers of the time also proffered their advice with regard to what must be done in the event of an outbreak of animal disease. In *The Boke of Husbandry*, John Fitzherbert, for example, wrote:

> And yf it fortune to fall murren amonge thy beastes, as god forbede, there be men ynough can helpe them. And it commeth of a ranknes of bloudde appereth most commonly fyrste in the heed: for his heed wyll swell, and his eyen waxe greate and ronne of water and frothe at the mouthe, and than he is paste remedy, and wyl dye shortely, and wyll neuer eate after he be sycke. Than slee hym, and make a depe pytte faste by, there as he dyeth, and caste hym in, and couer hym with erthe, that noo dogges maye come to the caryen, for as many beasts as feleth the smelle of that caryen, are lykely to be enfecte and take the skynne and haue it to the tanners to sell, and bryng it not home, for peryll that may fal. And it is commonly used, and commeth of a greate charytie, to take the bare heed of the same beaste, and put it on a longe pole, and set it in a hedge, faste bounden to a stake, ny the hyghe waye syde, that euery man, that rydethe or goeth that waye, maye se and knowe by that signe, that there is syckness of cattell in the townshyp.
>
> (Fitzherbert 1534: 35–6)

Heeding such advice and informing farming neighbours of cattle disease would doubtless have been important in preventing the further spread of disease. Throughout the seventeenth and eighteenth centuries, epizootics – most notably rinderpest, infectious bovine pleuropneumonia, foot-and-mouth disease and anthrax – continued to wreak havoc in Europe. During the early eighteenth century, the importation of livestock from Russia via Hungary to Italy brought rinderpest with it; such outbreaks often spread further westwards (Wilkinson 1992: 37–8). These outbreaks became increasingly well documented and continued to plague European livestock and human populations well into the nineteenth century.

The consequences of the increased movements of livestock throughout Europe during the eighteenth and nineteenth centuries will be explored in the following chapter in far greater detail. In the meantime, I will turn my attention to the kinds of measures taken to preserve animal health from antiquity to the early modern period. The following section will thus look at the emergence of animal medicine and early understandings of the nature and causes of animal disease.

The incipient veterinary regime

The inception of agrarianism in the Middle East – with its concomitant increased exploitation of and dependency on animal resources and the coming of animal plagues – also heralds the emergence of the veterinary regime. While one cannot speak of the existence of veterinary science or a veterinary profession *per se*, the period spanning from antiquity to the early modern period can be said to mark the first phase in the evolution of the veterinary regime. As domesticated animals became increasingly valuable to human societies, a need emerged to devote a degree of attention to their health and well-being. The process of intensive growth (i.e. the rise in the level of material comfort) – which in itself had been intensified by increasing animal use – ultimately made people more dependent on domesticated species to service their requirements (Jones 1988). Yet, at the same time, intensive growth had increased their need to take care of these animals and to deal with the diseases from which they suffered. Likewise, the process of extensive growth (i.e. increase in human population) precipitated the further intensification of animal use, thus necessitating people to turn their attention to the problem of animal health (Jones 1988). In order to ensure a continuous and healthy supply of animals, people were therefore compelled to develop the practical knowledge, skills and self-discipline necessary to maintain – an at least minimal level of – animal health; failing to do so would have seriously compromised agricultural productivity. As is also the case within modern farming practice, the onus of responsibility for the daily tending and feeding of animals generally lay with the animals' owners, or those either employed or enslaved to perform this task. However, from the earliest known civilisations onwards, specialists in the field of animal care and animal medicine began to emerge and offer their skills and services to animal owners.

In ancient Mesopotamia, the responsibility for protecting the health of animals fell specifically under the jurisdiction of priests; who claimed to be the mediators between the gods and their human servants. Ideas about illness were intimately tied to spiritual beliefs. Any disaster, such as disease, which befell was perceived as the result of the deity's displeasure. The priests maintained that the gods must continually be placated by obedience and sacrificial offerings, and when animal disease threatened, they would intervene to appease them. Thus a variety of specialists emerged to attend to the health needs of the ancient Mesopotamians and their animals. Through ritual sacrifice and the dissection of animal entrails, these priests recorded their detailed knowledge of animal pathology and anatomy in cuneiform texts and claimed responsibility for driving out the evil spirits that afflicted both humans and other animals with illness. More significantly, temple-based lay healers, known as *azus*, provided practical, rather than spiritual, help to the ancient Mesopotamian people and their animals. These specialists administered medicinal preparations and also practised surgery and obstetrics on their human and animal patients (Schwabe 1978: 103–5).

Likewise, in ancient Egypt, the burden of responsibility for animal care – particularly with regard to sacrificial animals – fell to the men of religion. Disease was believed to have supernatural origins, priests were therefore likely urged by animal owners to seek communion with the gods to ask them to intervene and preserve the health of ailing beasts. The early Egyptians' knowledge of the physiology and anatomy of animals – and through analogy that of humans – was inextricably interwoven with spiritual belief and religious ritual. Again, as in ancient Mesopotamia, there was a division of labour – particularly with regard to ritual duties – amongst different kinds of priest (Schwabe 1978: 72). It is thought that these priests probably gained much practical experience in looking after animals; the observations of animal biology which they made while performing their priestly rites – i.e. sacrifice and divination – were eventually translated into 'medical' knowledge which could be applied in the treatment of both animals and humans (Schwabe 1984: 256–7). This knowledge was transcribed by such priests. A few medical papyri, dating from the times of the Middle Kingdom, survived the passage of time and were unearthed during the late nineteenth century in archaeological excavations (Frey 1985). These papyri furnish us with concrete, though fragmentary, information about medical matters in ancient Egypt.

The Kahun papyrus is probably the most famous of these ancient

Egyptian medical texts and provides the most extensive detail on veterinary matters. Cattle diseases and their treatment feature prominently in this document, reflecting the religious and economic importance of this species to early Egyptian society. Besides cattle, the diseases of dogs, birds and fish are dealt with fragmentarily, concentrating largely on afflictions that concern the animal's eyes. The Kahun papyrus also contains a portion that appears to concern veterinary gynaecological matters (Schwabe 1978: 67). Egyptian art, pre-dating the Kahun papyrus by several centuries, also bears testimony to early Egyptian attempts at veterinary obstetrics. Tomb decorations, for example, depict animal attendants delivering calves by manual traction (Van der Weijden and Rozendal 1995: 81). Other Egyptian relics portray the removal of the placenta from cows and internal (rectal or vaginal) examinations of cattle (Schwabe 1978: 67). Ensuring a healthy supply of cattle's most important product – its offspring – was likely of great import to the ancient Egyptians, warranting the early development of veterinary obstetrics. Obstetricians, however, were not necessarily priests or lay healers, but could be specialist individuals holding titles such as the 'overseer of cattle' (Schwabe 1978: 79–80).

The shift from cattle to horse culture, as exemplified by ancient Greek and later Roman society, bore witness to a changing emphasis in animal medical specialisation. The Greek interest in horse and chariot racing and hunting fostered an erudite interest in equine medicine. Records, dating from around 500 BC, show that specialist horse doctors (*hippiatros*) existed in Ancient Greek society, being employed by many city states. It is, however, thought that these *hippiatros* sometimes practised their art on cattle, sheep, pigs and dogs, in addition to horses (Schwabe 1978: 127). Accounts reveal that relatively complex surgery was performed on animals at this time; special constraining devices having been invented so that large animals could be operated on. In large cities, *zooiatreions*, which housed such apparatus, were opened for the treatment of sick animals (Karasszon 1988: 70). The use of such animal hospitals was, however, likely reserved for the treatment of the prized horses of the wealthy. Agricultural folk were unlikely to have had access to (or be aware of) such facilities and the knowledge of the great physicians. Instead, they were more likely to have relied on experience, techniques and elixirs developed over generations through trial and error, rather than recent scientific developments.

As Bodson (1994) suggests, ancient breeders and animal doctors were not scientists at all, but were instead effective managers who were sensitive to the animal's state of well-being and based their cures on experience, rather than on theories of disease. Consequently, these empirics were able, through observation, to recognise the detrimental effects of (visible) disease-causing parasites such as worms and insects, without recourse to the theories on the origins of disease which the urban philosopher-physicians advanced (Bodson 1994: 305). Bodson has in fact concluded that throughout classical antiquity animal medicine remained 'primarily a matter of empirical practice, never reaching any level comparable to that of Aristotelian zoology or human medicine of the Hippocratic school' (Bodson 1996: 1592). Yet while the ancient animal doctors may not have attained a level of theoretical development equivalent to their human medical counterparts, Greek thinkers and physicians nonetheless had a significant influence on the ideas and (veterinary) medical practice of future generations. Indeed, as we shall see in the following chapter, the disease concept of humoral pathology – i.e. the notion (espoused by Hippocrates amongst others) that disease results from the affection of the body's fluids – remained influential to veterinary medicine until the nineteenth century AD.

In the largely agrarian-based society of ancient Rome, animal medicine was the general preserve of livestock holders who relied on their own practical experience and folk knowledge to treat the animals on which they depended, rather than that of specialist physicians. As Karasszon puts it, 'when the Greek medicine had reached its golden age, there were no physicians in Rome and curing relied on the use of domestic remedies like wine and cabbage-prickling [sic] brine' (Karasszon 1988: 85). Roman medicine thus relied greatly on practical experience, traditional remedies and appeals to household gods to deliver family, slaves and livestock from plague. When Greek physicians began to come to Rome to practise their medical art, they were initially treated with great suspicion, discredited or even exiled (Smithcors 1957: 59). Hellenic influence, however, eventually prevailed, as the works of the Greek philosopher-physicians were read and translated into Latin and their ideas about human and animal health and remedies were adopted or adapted by the Romans. There was, however, a great divide between medical scientific knowledge and everyday practice. Roman patricians studied and versed themselves in the medical texts of their Greek examples, but medical practice was generally considered too base a profession and they gained scant tangible experience in dealing with human sickness and disease

(Karasszon 1988: 91). Treating food-producing animals then most certainly belonged to the realm of agriculture, rather than cultivated urban life.

It is therefore the Roman agricultural writers who offer the greatest detail on the way in which disease was dealt with in Ancient Roman society. Cato the Elder, the most famous of these, presented a straightforward solution to the problem of disease. Putting profit above all else, he advised owners of diseased animals (and slaves) to simply sell them off to the highest bidder or, if this failed, to drive them into the wilderness before they became a burden (Wilkinson 1992: 8). In sharp contrast, Varro, a later agricultural writer, had a more enlightened approach to the care of livestock. In his work *De Re Rustica*, he placed a strong emphasis on the necessity of feeding, breeding, raising and maintaining the health of domesticated animals, recognising that sickness in just a single animal could spell disaster for the entire herd and, as a consequence, the farmer's economic position (Hooper and Ash 1934). Moreover, while Varro advocates that the farmer or animal attendant should learn and practise the art of animal healing, he does allude to the existence of specialist animal doctors who should be called in if surgery is required (Hooper and Ash 1934). Although Varro's ideas about the causes of disease bear strong resemblance to the Hippocratic notions of humoral pathology – evidencing the growing influence of Greek medicine in the Roman world – he does in fact speculate on the possibility of disease-causing microorganisms. In advising farmers not to locate their farms near swamps and marshy areas, he writes that

> there are bred certain minute creatures which cannot be seen by the eyes, which float in the air and enter the body through the mouth and nose and there cause serious diseases.
>
> (Hooper and Ash 1934: 209)

Varro's conjecture about the existence of such 'animalculae', as he goes on to describe them, suggests that he thought contagion to be an important factor in coping with disease. In this regard, he advocated certain measures that would prevent the spread of disease amongst herds and flocks. For example, he recommends the isolation of sick and pregnant animals in separate enclosures (Hooper and Ash 1934: 339) and keeping several smaller herds of goats in several locations, rather than in one big group, to prevent disease from spreading quickly and ruining the farmer (Hooper and Ash 1934: 34–5). Some fifty years later, Columella also addressed the topic of contagion and quarantine; with respect to oxen he cautioned his readers that they

> must also beware, that neither a sow nor a hen creep into their cribs; for that which fall for them, being mixed with their fodder, is certain death to oxen; and that especially, which a sick sow throws up and vomits, is enough to raise a plague; and when this lights on a herd, you must presently change the climate, and, having distributed the cattle into several divisions, you must go with them into regions that lie at a great distance; and the diseased must be separated from the sound, that not so much as one may come among them, which may, with the contagion, infect the rest. Therefore, when they are removed to a great distance, they must be brought into those places wherein no other cattle are fed, lest, by their coming, they bring the plague also among them.
>
> (Columella 1745: 265)

Such ideas about contagion were hardly expanded on for another eighteen centuries, after which time 'germ theory' – as will be illustrated in the following chapter – eventually became a favoured explanation of disease. Besides Columella's and Varro's contributions, little else was actually written about animal disease prevention through the adoption of quarantine measures until long after the Middle Ages (Smithcors 1957: 67). With regard to the understanding of disease transmission, it was only Galen who further contributed to the notion of contagion. Akin to Varro, he used the expression 'seeds of disease', in relation to contagion and infectious disease, to draw an analogy between what he observed in the natural world around him and the unknown and invisible which, he postulated, caused disease (Nutton 1983).

Equine medicine

As in ancient Greece, the specialist animal doctors within Roman society seem to have largely restricted their practice to the treatment and care of equine species. Indeed, the importance of horses to support military regimes could confer considerable status on those who treated them. The earliest Latin term for a horse doctor, dating from around the end of the first century BC, was *equarius medicus* (Bodson 1996: 1592). Later, the term *mulomedicus* (mule doctor) was more commonly used to describe those who healed horses and other equids (Walker 1973: 314). *Mulomedici* were hereditary public slaves who were responsible for dealing with the injuries of the animals employed by the imperial postal transport services. Roman animal doctors, however, came from many social strata; some were indeed slaves, but others were freedmen or military men (Fischer 1988: 192–3). Other names such as *medicus veterinarius*, *medicus iumentarius* and *medicus pecuarius* (livestock doctor) were occasionally employed in the late Roman empire to describe animal doctors; the first epithet was bestowed on higher ranking army personnel (Bodson 1996: 1592).

It was to be the horse doctors of the Roman world who would set the trend for the future of animal medicine; until the mid-eighteenth century the practice of animal medicine was to be more or less equatable with equine medicine (Schwabe 1978). From Roman times onwards, a body of specialist knowledge on the health, diseases and management of horses was gradually built up. For example, during the late fourth century AD, the Roman author Vegetius Renatus compiled a work entitled the *Mulomedicina* which was devoted to the diseases of horses and mules (Walker 1973: 303). Particularly within the Byzantine Empire – which lasted until 1453, long after the decline and fall of the western part of the Roman Empire – there were also significant advances in the understanding of equine care and conditions (Doyen-Higuet 1984). During the tenth century AD, Byzantine knowledge of equine medicine was eventually collected and compiled into a single volume, the *Hippiatrica.* This text provided the foundation of written knowledge on the topic for centuries to come; particularly after having been translated from its Greek original to Latin in 1530 (Dunlop and Williams 1996: 185).

Horses continued to play an ever-increasingly important role in European society throughout the Middle Ages. The invention of nailed-on horseshoes greatly improved the performance of cavalry and draught horses, and their use spread throughout Europe during the early Middle Ages. Likewise, metallurgical technology was employed to produce stirrups that would enable riders to remain on horseback more easily; thus increasing the effectiveness of cavalry still further (Clutton-Brock 1992: 73–6). The care of the cavalry horses which participated in military campaigns, in addition to the maintenance of the nobility's hunting steeds and later those mounts that took part in religious crusades, became an increasingly important preoccupation and required the skills of specialists. In the royal courts, horse marshals were appointed to service the horses of the aristocracy. Essentially, such men were horse trainers who possessed a practical knowledge of the management and care of the equine species. However, treating these esteemed animals in health and disease was also their responsibility. One of the most renowned of these mediaeval marshals was Jordanus Ruffus, who was appointed to the court of Frederick II (1194–1250). At his patron's behest, Ruffus produced a work on equine medicine that would go on to serve as a manual for horse users and tenders for many centuries to come (Dunlop and Williams 1996: 225).

During the sixteenth and seventeenth centuries, horse marshals continued to impart their wisdom with regard to the training and management of horses. For example, in 1550 the Italian horse trainer Frederick Grisone published the *Rules for Riding*, a text that featured rather ruthless and punitive methods to get horses to acquiesce to their human masters. In England too, similar texts appeared that were devoted to all aspects of horse-riding, breaking, breeding, management and cure (e.g. Browne 1620, 1624). Another of these celebrated horse marshals was Jacques Labessie de Solleysel. His book *Le Parfait Maréchal* (1664), which dealt with horse management and disease, became immensely popular and underwent numerous reprints, being translated into both German and English. Veterinary historians regard De Solleysel as an important contributor to the understanding of the nature of equine disease because he recognised the contagiousness of conditions such as strangles and glanders. Marshals were held in particularly high regard by their royal or aristocratic employers and were accorded a great deal of prestige. Their skills at teaching horsemanship became increasingly important to the ruling elite of European society as the horse continued to grow in significance for warfare, even after technological innovations such as cannons and guns had entered into the fray (Dunlop and Williams 1996: 262, 272).

The work of marshals, however, appears to have been restricted to the royal courts that employed them. During mediaeval times and throughout the early modern period, the medical care of horses was generally entrusted either to the blacksmiths who shoed them, or to farriers. Farriers in particular assumed the burden of responsibility for equine health; though unlike the high-ranking horse marshals, they have generally been portrayed as being uneducated and of a lowly social class (Pugh 1962: 4). Indeed, farriers appear to have had a notorious reputation for their ignorance. As cavalry captain William Burden wrote in his 1730 publication *The Gentleman's Pocket Farrier*:

> A Farrier is as useful a trade as any other in His majesty's Dominions; we commonly call him Doctor, because he professes Physick and Surgery among horse; and some are good sensible Men, but people who are able to give their Sons learning, seldom bind 'em to that trade; so that Farriers are obliged to take such Apprentices as they can get, without regard to their Education. When an Apprentice has served out his Time, a few Recipe's (the same that for Time out of Mind have secretly been handed down from Master to Man, without any Variation or Amendment) set him up; and fully contented, he seeks to know no more: Thus many are illiterate and some totally incapable of improvement.
>
> (Hall 1991: 10)

John Lawrence, a later author who penned *A Philosophical and Practical Treatise on Horses and the Moral Duties of Man Towards the Brute Creation* (1796), was even more scathing on the treatment that horses received from both owners and farriers during the seventeenth and early eighteenth centuries:

> The wretched, ill-fated animal, after having been maimed and crippled in the service of his unrelenting master, was consigned to additional and useless torture under the hands of an ignorant and brutal farrier, who mangled his devoted limbs with senseless and inapplicable operations, or drenched his body with nauseous and unmeaning slops; of the merits of which, the judgement of the doctor and his patient were nearly on a level. The broth of fodden whelps, dogs t—d and wine, chickens guts, human ordure fresh from the alembic . . . numbered among the choicest of veterinary specifics.
>
> (Lawrence 1796: 24–5)

Farriers were popularly depicted by eighteenth-century cartoonists as being 'grossly incompetent, crude and cruel in [their] methods and rapacious' (Pugh 1962: 4). Their misguidedness was in part put down by later authors to their ignorance of disease and the structure and workings of the animal body (Pattison 1984: 1). However, much of the blame has been apportioned to the influential writings and remedies of one man: Gervase Markham. A self-styled expert on matters of animal medicine, horsemanship and husbandry, Markham (1562–1637) was a highly prolific and successful author. Many of his works, such as *Markham's Maister-Peece* (1610), ran to numerous editions and were still in popular use for more than a century after his death; although he is commonly portrayed by later authors as a dangerous charlatan. Lawrence, for instance, describes him as 'the oracle of sapient grooms, the fiddle of old wives, and the glory of booksellers'. He goes on to claim that the extensive circulation of Markham's work 'brought about as many evils and cruel inflictions on poor helpless animals, as the opening of Pandora's box did on the human race' (Lawrence 1796: 11). Lawrence continues with a harsh warning to his contemporaries:

> From the works of Gervase Markham, and his famous receipts, all the old grooms and farriers, who (unfortunately for the animals committed to their care, and the proprietors of them, were able to read and write) obtained all their veterinary knowledge, their skill in operations, and their wonderful tricks; nor is the fame of this great writer altogether unknown to some of our elder sages of the stable, even this day; and I must be leave to advise every owner of horses, who regards their welfare and his own interest, as soon as he shall be apprised of Markham's works, or indeed any of that stamp, to purchase such dangerous commodities out of their hands; and to put them to more harmless and necessary purposes, than to those to which ignorant people would most probably apply them.
>
> (Lawrence 1796:11)

Not all seventeenth- and eighteenth-century farriers and writers on equine medicine, however, were tarred with the same brush as Markham. William Hope's *The Compleat Horseman* (1680), a translation of De Solleysel's famous work, was seen as a great advance for the care and treatment of horses. During the first half of the eighteenth century, several works on the art of farriery appeared that were penned by human surgeons, who often had substantial (military) experience with or an interest in treating horses (e.g. Bracken 1738; Gibson 1738). It has recently been suggested that our modern perception of the social standing and competence of farriers during the eighteenth century is largely inaccurate.

Farriers, argues Joan Lane (1993), have persistently been depicted in veterinary historical literature as illiterate and low-grade artisans, often having been confused with blacksmiths. There is, she asserts, much evidence, e.g. bills, receipts, partnership agreements, employment contracts and occasionally even publications, to suggest that they were mostly far from unlettered and, moreover, that they were highly valued by their wealthier clients who relied on them to tend their valuable racehorses and other mounts. Lane contends that the modern view of farriery has generally been based on the views of those, such as Lawrence (1796), who condemned the trade some 200 years ago, largely for their own ends. In this context, she makes an interesting comparison with the nineteenth-century poor law reformers in Britain who, to improve their chances of overturning the existing legal statutes, denigrated the poor law to make their own views more acceptable (Lane 1993: 110–12). Such critics were indeed successful for, as the next chapter will illustrate, during the second half of the eighteenth century, the medical care of horses was gradually taken out of the hands of farriers and became the eventual responsibility of college-educated veterinary surgeons.

Understanding and curing animal disease

Neither the farriers nor the horse marshals would have been of much real use to animal owners in the advent of infectious disease; although they certainly proffered many remedies and claimed numerous cures for it. Since ancient times, one disease in particular posed a significant threat to horse populations and consequently to both the economic and military activities of human society. Glanders – or farcy as its cutaneous form was known, often being regarded as a separate disease – also presented considerable risks to human health, although – as will be illustrated in the next chapter – its zoonotic nature was only recognised in the early nineteenth century. There was a considerable difference of opinion when it came to the issue of its contagiousness. Ruffus, for example, recommended that glanderous horses should be put to graze with others 'in order to get rid of their discharges'; whereas De Solleysel firmly believed that sick horses should be segregated at the earliest hint of the disease and prevented from sharing the same drinking troughs as healthy ones (Blancou 1994: 412). From ancient times onwards, attempts were made to keep this disease under surveillance and to control it through segregation, and even the slaughter of diseased horses. The treatment of glanders through surgical excision, cauterisation, castration, bleeding and prayer was also attempted throughout mediaeval times and during the early modern period (Blancou ibid.: 414).

While glanders posed a clear threat to the horses that were essential for transportation, draught and warfare, food-producing animals continued to be struck by terrible animal plagues. As the above discussion suggests, these epizootics could put the agricultural economy in jeopardy. Again, people were fairly helpless in the event of animal plagues. During the mediaeval and early modern periods, there was very little advancement in understanding of animal disease and its transmission. By the thirteenth century, there had been a revival of interest in the study of science and medicine, particularly within monastic orders such as the Dominicans and Franciscans. Universities began to spring up around Europe during the late Middle Ages, providing new centres of learning. Further to this, the crusades to Palestine engendered a resurgence of interest in matters of animal medicine, particularly within Italy, as Arabian horses and knowledge of Arab horsemanship were brought back from the east; though, as Lise Wilkinson observes, the movements of troops and animals brought epizootics in their wake (Wilkinson 1992: 18–22). However, even with this regenerated interest, people still continued to rely on the teachings of the ancients, which had either been translated into Latin or compiled and expounded on by mediaeval encyclopaedists such as Albertus Magnus. Even into the seventeenth century, the wisdom and remedies of the ancients can be found entwined with contemporary beliefs and superstitions about the causes and cures of animal disease in well-known texts such as Edward Topsell's *The Historie of Foure-Footed Beastes* (1607).

During the Middle Ages, people were inclined to rely on amulets, relics and incantations to protect or cure their livestock from disease (Dunlop and Williams 1996: 235). One can find evidence of this in the literature of the time. In the prologue to Chaucer's *Pardoner's Tale*, for instance, his protagonist produces sheep's shoulder-bone which is claimed to be a holy relic that has great prophylactic powers for animals (Blake 1980: 439). Mystical animal healers proliferated during the mediaeval period, the most famous of which was St Hildegard, a Benedictine nun who recommended a wide range of herbal treatments for both human and animal disease and employed her religious powers and amulets to cure. Onyx stones, for instance, were used in the treatment of plagues (Dunlop and Williams 1996: 215). Next to these mystics, there was another class of itinerant specialists who employed their skills in the treatment of animals. Cow-leeches, as these men were known, relied on blood-letting and a range of herbal remedies to treat animal disease, and were ubiquitously found throughout rural society from mediaeval times onwards. Gervase Markham (1648) provides an example of the kind of remedy that was probably employed by seventeenth-century leeches to treat cattle plague and contemporary understandings of its causes:

> Murraine amongst beasts is bred by divers occasions; as from ranknesse of bloud, or feeding, from corruption of the ayre, intemperateness of the weather, inundation of flouds, or the infection of other *Cattel*: much might be said of the violence and mortality thereof, which utterly unfurnished whole Countries; but to go to the cure, *you shall give to all your cattel, as wel the sound as sick, this medicine, which never failed to preserve as many as have taken it:* take of old urine a quart, and mixe it with a handfull of Hens dung dissolved therein, and leat your beast drink it.
>
> (Markham 1648: 96)

Cow-leeches are regarded somewhat acrimoniously by later authors as being the lowest common denominator within animal medicine. Pugh (1962), for instance, writes of how the herds of prized cattle that were bred with great care during the eighteenth century were 'abandoned to the care of the cow-leech'. At best, he claims, 'the cow-leeches probably did nothing to prevent the recovery of their patients by natural means; at worst, they certainly inflicted unnecessary pain' (Pugh 1962: 3). Because the cow leech tended to rely on traditional remedies that were by this time well known to the literate, Pugh suggests that many leeches came to depend on amulets, charms and incantations to keep the confidence of their humbler clients. Occasionally, he contends, they even went so far as to partake in ceremonies where cattle were burnt or buried alive. As the following chapter will illustrate, cow-leeches persisted well into the nineteenth century and continued to practise their art in the face of the rise of rational medicine (Pugh ibid.: 4).

By the close of the fifteenth century, a more erudite interest in both human and animal medicine began to emerge. The study of (comparative) anatomy was increasingly undertaken, finding artistic expression in, amongst others, the work of Leonardo da Vinci

(Dunlop and Williams 1996: 237–58). The renaissance in science was centred in Italy, just as the renaissance in art and architecture had been in the second half of the fourteenth century (Wilkinson 1992: 24). During the mid-sixteenth century, scientific attention turned once again to the notion of contagion. The concept of 'seeds of disease' that had been expressed by Galen centuries earlier was echoed by Girolamo Fracastoro in *De Contagione* (1546) (Brock 1961: 69–75); this text is thought to be the very first treatise specifically devoted to the contagious diseases of both animals and humans (Nutton 1983). Wilkinson (1992) suggests that Fracastoro may have found inspiration for this work in the devastating outbreaks of foot-and-mouth disease that swept through his homeland at the time. Like other authors who went before him, Fracastoro also recognised the necessity of isolating infected animals from the herd. Later, during the mid-seventeenth century, Fracastoro's ideas were developed further by Athanasius Kircher, who advanced the notion that the agents responsible for disease may indeed be living organisms. By the end of the century, Antonie van Leeuwenhoek had proved the existence of animalcules through his self-made microscope, in this regard speculating also on cattle disease (Brock 1961: 8–11). Leeuwenhoek's discovery, Wilkinson suggests, along with the increasing concern for the cattle epizootics that continued to threaten the agricultural economy throughout Europe, may have made some inroads into changing contemporary scientific thought on disease causation; which until then had revolved almost exclusively around the notion of spontaneous generation (Wilkinson 1992: 26–30).

Cattle plague continued to have a major impact on European society into the eighteenth century. During the second decade of the century, a major epizootic of rinderpest swept throughout the continent, apparently following in the path of the Swedish and Russian armies. This plague claimed around 1.5 million cattle within five years and spread to all corners of Europe, even crossing the Channel to the British Isles by 1714 (Dunlop and Williams 1996: 279). The cattle plague was particularly rampant in Italy in 1711 and progressively devastated the national livestock population. As Wilkinson (1984) observes, although cattle plagues had sporadically occurred throughout the seventeenth century, they had been largely overshadowed by the great plague epidemics that had been faced by humans. People were quite unprepared to face epizootics on this scale. The cattle plague persisted and within months of its initial outbreak, the Venetian authorities appealed to the medical faculty at Padua for help (Wilkinson ibid.: 131). The faculty's principal Bernardino Ramazzini came to their aid, making several proposals with regard to the possible control of the plague through the employment of hygienic measures, isolation of infected animals and the fumigation of stalls. Rejecting astrological explanations of disease, he forwarded the idea that rinderpest was spread through contagion, in so doing comparing the course of the disease with that of smallpox in humans (Wilkinson ibid.: 132). In this regard, Ramazzini also attempted to apply the principle of variolation, which had previously been used to prevent smallpox, to protect cattle against the plague (Dunlop and Williams 1996: 279). Ramazzini was eventually joined in his appeals to take adequate measures against the cattle plague by fellow physician, Giovanni Maria Lancisi. Lancisi wrote more extensively on cattle plague and, perhaps because he was the personal physician to the Pope, the authorities – although offering a degree of resistance and reluctance – eventually took heed of his advice and implemented quarantine, isolation and slaughter measures, thus leading to the control of the outbreak (Wilkinson 1984: 133). Lancisi's method of dealing with cattle disease through the systematic slaughter of all sick animals and those suspected of harbouring the disease proved to be the most effective means of control. In 1714, the Englishman Thomas Bates proposed a similarly strict system of control, and the further spread of cattle plague throughout Britain was curtailed within a matter of months. This method of animal disease control was also successfully employed in other parts of Europe, such as the Austrian Netherlands (Bieleman 1992: 163).

The epizootics of the eighteenth century clearly highlighted the dearth of scientific knowledge about animal disease and the dangers it posed to the agricultural economy. Moreover, the coming of such plagues demonstrated the inefficacy of the existing veterinary regime. Ramazzini's and Lancisi's interest in the cattle plague, however, marks an important turning point for the study and control of animal disease. These Italian physicians were able to demonstrate that the discussion of animal disease was indeed not beneath the dignity of medical men. With such respectable medical attentions being directed towards it, the study of animal disease finally began to receive a degree of scientific legitimisation (Wilkinson 1992: 46). In the following chapter, we shall see how the veterinary regime entered its second and most crucial phase and went on to gain much greater legitimisation in the wake of much greater cattle plagues and far newer scientific understandings.

4

THE UNFOLDING VETERINARY REGIME

Introduction

Until the mid-eighteenth century, European society had been based predominantly on agrarianism. Agriculture and animal husbandry provided the mainstay of the European economy and the means with which the vast majority could survive, often on a hand-to-mouth basis. Within agrarian society, people tended to live in very close proximity with domesticated animals and were dependent on those animals for their everyday subsistence. It was not unusual that farmers and their families lived together with their livestock under one roof. The house and byre were often combined, separated only by a wall or cross passage. Even townsfolk would attempt to keep poultry, pigs and even cattle in their backyards and bedrooms in order to procure a regular supply of milk, eggs and some meat for the winter months. In this regard, Keith Thomas notes that cows were milked in city streets and, for many centuries, 'pigs were a notorious hazard of urban life', starting fires, biting people and even killing small children (Thomas 1983: 94–5). Needless to say, the close proximity in which humans and animals lived provided considerable opportunities for the transmission of infectious diseases across the species' divide.

The agrarian character of European society was, however, to be transformed as people began to develop new ideas and technologies and to tap the natural energy resources offered by fossil fuels. Industrialisation was to be the third major ecological transition exacted by humans. As Johan Goudsblom has observed, like the domestication of fire and agrarianisation before it, industrialisation involved 'the incorporation into human society of natural forces that were previously outside the human realm' (1992: 164). The process of industrialisation was a gradual one, occurring at different rates and intensity within the individual nations of Europe, depending on the peculiarities of the social, political and economic circumstances of each country. Traditionally it is Britain that has been given the pride of place as the cradle of industrialisation. From the late eighteenth century onwards, the nation underwent a remarkable transition from agricultural to industrial production. This transition was accompanied by a tremendous rate of both extensive and intensive growth. The size of the population grew rapidly and the levels of material comfort rose substantially as Britain became increasingly industrialised. By the mid-nineteenth century, the impact of the industrialisation process could be felt throughout the society as a whole. Yet while the industrialisation process in Britain was in full swing, the transition to industrial production in neighbouring countries had barely begun; although it is fair to say that certain industrial innovations and technologies were embraced and employed without a country necessarily yet having undergone the process of industrialisation. In the Netherlands, the industrialisation process only started around 1870 – some 90 years later than in Britain – and only really picked up speed after 1890.

Although there were great disparities in the time and place that industrialisation took place, it is fair to conclude that the result was ultimately the same, for, in each country, the process of industrialisation led to significant and irreversible social change. The increasing urbanisation of society was one of the major consequences of industrialisation; though it is worth noting that the Netherlands had already become significantly urbanised by the end of the eighteenth century as a result of earlier commercial development (de Vries 1984). Yet even there, as in Britain, people increasingly flocked to towns and cities in order to seek their fortunes and gain employment in the new factories that had been established there. The introduction of land enclosure contributed to this migration as people were driven off the land and needed to seek employment elsewhere. Once the dual processes of industrialisation and urbanisation had got under way, it was not long before commerce and manufacturing overtook agriculture as the primary source of wealth. With mass migration to urban areas, the number of people involved in agriculture and animal husbandry steadily declined; yet, at the same time, the – increasingly predominantly urban – population continued to expand, leading to ever-increasing food demands and consequently to an intensification of animal use. The radical transformation of western European society precipitated a significant change in the relationship between humans and other animals. No longer involved in the daily trials and tribulations of rural life, the ever-expanding urban populace neither came into regular contact with agricultural animals, nor were they directly economically dependent on them for their livelihood.

These social changes were also reflected in a significant transformation in attitudes towards animals. From the eighteenth century onwards, diminishing contact with animals meant that the urban population were far removed from the harsh realities of the human–animal relationship. This coincided with more general changes in the personality structure of individuals, which had led to a greatly heightened 'delicacy of feeling', particularly amongst the bourgeoisie. As Norbert Elias (1994) argued, the transformation of the psychological make-up of individuals was a consequence of the changing social relations that occurred alongside state formation and the monopolisation of organised violence during the early modern period. These changing sensibilities were exemplified by a growing aversion to brutality and social or physical contamination, in addition to an increasing sense of defencelessness and greater propensity to experience embarrassment, shame and repugnance, most particularly with regard to bodily functions and disease (Goudsblom 1986). More importantly, these changes in personality structure implied new thresholds in self and social control and more differentiated patterns of conduct. The growing sensitivity to both witnessing and performing violent acts found expression in the emergence of a bourgeois humanitarian movement – the antecedent of today's animal rights crusade – which lamented and protested against cruelty to animals. A further consequence of such changing sensibilities was that the routine slaughter of animals was banished from the immediate view of the middle classes and pushed behind the scenes of society, slaughterhouses being situated only on the fringes of urban areas where they could not offend or remind the sensitive of the origins of their food (Koolmees 1997).

The estrangement of the urban population from the realities of agricultural life also removed them from the immediate (economic) effects of animal disease. Yet it was at this time that serious epizootics raged across Europe claiming livestock victims in their hundreds of thousands. Animal plagues, such as rinderpest, pleuropneumonia and foot-and-mouth disease, posed a great threat to the wealth and health of European nations during the late eighteenth and nineteenth centuries. And, as will shortly be illustrated, it was the changing nature and composition of the emergent industrial society that in part contributed to the coming of these plagues. This chapter primarily explores the consequences of these epizootics for western European society, in the light of the social and historical changes that took place during this period. It will look at how such animal plagues and other social, economic and intellectual factors influenced the gradual formalisation and intensification of the veterinary regime within Europe. The first part will thus examine the establishment of formal veterinary education and the birth of a true veterinary profession; the second explores the emergent role of the state in dealing with epizootic disease and protecting the agricultural economy. Governmental responses to outbreaks of cattle plague in Britain and the Netherlands during the nineteenth century will form the basis of this discussion.

The birth of the veterinary profession

For many centuries, as the previous chapter illustrated, the care and treatment of animals rested generally in the hands of farriers and cow-leeches, in addition to those of the animal's owners themselves. By the late eighteenth century, these animal doctors increasingly came to be criticised by contemporaries for their gross incompetence, cruelty to animals and the crudity of their methods (Pugh 1962). Their supposed notoriety was such that one modern commentator has gone so far as to draw the conclusion that 'the most fortunate sick animals in the 18th century were those left untreated. Their companions bled, purged, blistered, and fired, suffered and died' (Pattison 1984: 2). It seems, however, that this statement echoes the sentiments of the past, for it was during the mid-eighteenth century that the first decisive steps were taken to remove the medical treatment and care from the hands of these purportedly brutal and socially inferior empirics and to place it in those of trained and 'scientifically educated' men.

Several factors were influential in this development. The first of these that may be identified is the changing intellectual climate in this period, which had led to a more general shift from tradition to reason and from magic to science. John Fisher (1995) has argued that the veterinary profession is a child born of the 'age of reason'; a clear product of the ascent of a new kind of science that was based on observation, experimentation and inductive reasoning. The new scientific mentality that developed during the Enlightenment, Fisher suggests, was also responsible for a reappraisal of nature, which led to a great transformation in the perception of people's relationship with other animals and a growing curiosity for studying them (Fisher ibid.: 45). As we have already seen in the introduction to this book, it was within this intellectual climate that new theological and philosophical notions of humankind being the caretakers of the natural world, rather than controllers of it, emerged. The pursuit of knowledge became increasingly important during the eighteenth century as people sought to understand the workings of the world in which they lived. Education, as Fisher contends, provided the key to acquiring, transmitting and effectively using such knowledge. The veterinary schools that were established across western Europe during the latter half of the eighteenth century are exemplary of this trend of upholding the 'sovereignty of knowledge', though, as Fisher points out, it was to be a long time before the activities of the new veterinary profession were to be truly shaped by the tenets of science. For while veterinary education was to be couched in such terms, tradition – as will shortly be discussed – continued to prevail in the practical treatment of animals (Fisher ibid.: 45–6).

A second factor that strongly influenced attempts to create a new and more effective brand of animal doctor was the increasingly devastating impact of animal plagues on livestock production. As the previous chapter illustrated, since 1709 the agricultural economy had been repeatedly under attack from a terrible new cattle plague, issuing from the eastern Steppe region, which threatened to wipe out the cattle population. This cattle plague, known as contagious typhoid fever, steppe murrain and later by its modern name rinderpest, was responsible for the decimation of livestock and the financial ruin of farmers. For example, in the years 1713–19, 1744–59 and 1768–86, the Dutch cattle population and agricultural community were struck and devastated by such animal plagues. The empirics provided no reliable answers or effective cures; essentially all people felt they could do was to pray and beg the Lord to put an end to their ordeal (Offringa 1976: 164). By 1744, after relatively successful endeavours to prevent smallpox through the technique of variolation, attempts to inoculate animals against rinderpest in a similar fashion were made in Britain and the Netherlands (Offringa 1983: 416). This method involved material extracted from an infected animal being inserted into a healthy one through surgical incisions. Variolation in cattle, however, seems to have been far less successful than it had been in humans (Dunlop and Williams 1996: 408). After a serious outbreak of the disease in 1799, the inoculation of cattle in such a fashion came to be banned in the Netherlands on 'penalty of flogging and banishment'

(Kerstens 1971: 13). While these epizootics continued to rage throughout Europe, other infectious diseases such as glanders, anthrax and sheep-pox also wreaked havoc amongst animal populations and within human society (Offringa 1983: 414–15). National governments, increasingly concerned with their country's economic prosperity and the problems that the agricultural world was suffering, gradually began to sit up and take notice of the social and economic impact of animal disease and the necessity of attacking the problem in a systematic and scientific fashion.

The establishment of veterinary schools

It was in France that the first governmental moves towards dealing with the problem of animal disease through science and education were made. In 1762, the very first *école pour le traitement des maladies des bestiaux* was set up in Lyon by Claude Bourgelat, a lawyer by training and the stable-master of the city's riding school, with the financial support of his friend, Henri-Léonard Bertin, general inspector of finances and a minister in the government of Louis XV (Ballarini and Ferrando 1988; Loew 1990). According to Offringa, both men were deeply affected by the devastation that the cattle plague had left in its wake and the necessity of acquiring greater knowledge on animal disease. But it was Bertin who was to insist that the school they were to set up would devote itself to more than just the study of equine medicine; which had, as the previous chapter suggested, been more or less the sole focus of inquiry into animal health in centuries past (Offringa 1983: 415). Equine medicine, however, continued to play an important role within the veterinary school, for the military required increasing numbers of horses for its activities and people competent and skilled enough to care for them properly (Ballarini and Ferrando 1988). Within three years, Bourgelat had established a second *école vétérinaire* at Alfort, close to Paris. At this school, students learned the practical skills of shoeing horses, in addition to receiving a theoretical education covering a diverse range of subjects, such as anatomy, botany, zoology, pharmacy, therapy, surgery, legal veterinary studies, animal husbandry and animal care. Bourgelat was particularly keen to enrol the sons of smiths for he considered them the best candidates for the study and practice of animal medicine. The veterinary school at Alfort became the model on which future veterinary schools in Europe were to be based. Similar veterinary schools were to be established in

Copenhagen (1773), Vienna (1777), Hannover (1778), Dresden (1780), Munich (1790), Berlin (1790) and Utrecht (1820). A veterinary college was set up in London (1791), which, although inspired by the French example, had a character quite different to its counterparts on mainland Europe (Offringa 1983: 415).

The case of the London Veterinary College is a particularly interesting one for it was a privately funded enterprise, rather than one that derived its income from the state. The idea of establishing such a college for veterinary education in Britain was the brainchild of the, otherwise historically obscure, Agricultural Society of Odiham in the southerly county of Hampshire. During the latter half of the eighteenth century, such upper-class organisations dedicated to promoting the 'improvement' of agriculture proliferated throughout Britain, acting in many respects as 'proxies' for the state in all matters agricultural (Fisher 1995: 47). Aware of developments in neighbouring France, the Society concluded in 1785 that 'farriery is a most useful science and intimately connected with the interests of agriculture; that is in a very imperfect neglected state and highly deserving the attention of all friends of the agricultural economy' (Pattison 1984: 2). The Society thus devised a plan to establish a veterinary college in London, following the French example. These plans eventually came to fruition and in 1792 the doors of the School finally opened to its fee-paying students, who began a three-year residential course of instruction based largely on equine studies, though with some instruction on the 'epizootic diseases of farm animals' included in the curriculum. Charles Vial de St Bel, a graduate veterinarian of the Lyon school whose help had been enlisted in setting up the School, was appointed as the new School's professor (Pattison 1984; Porter 1993).

As the Odiham Agricultural Society had been keen to recognise, developments within the British agricultural sector during this period necessitated increased attention to matters of animal health. The late eighteenth century bore witness to the commencement of a transition from labour-intensive to capital-intensive farming, that would eventually culminate – as the next chapter will discuss in detail – in the industrialisation of agricultural production. The shift to capital-intensive farming was more prevalent at that time in Britain than in other parts of western Europe. This change was to be typified by the livestock sector, where increasing numbers of animals were being kept to meet increasing consumer demands for animal produce, yet where the numbers of people involved in managing those animals were on the decline. Livestock were becoming increasingly valuable to farmers and their value needed to be protected; this created an important market for the services of specialist veterinarians who could satisfy livestock producers' needs (Fisher 1995: 47). Likewise, as Fisher points out, this growing market for veterinary services was also reflected within the transport sector, for at this time there was a steady growth in coaching services requiring a constant supply of healthy and disease-free horses to pull carriages (Fisher ibid.).

Alongside these late-eighteenth-century developments – that brought about an increased market for the services of veterinary specialists – came a change in military organisation and strategy that would necessitate the skills of properly trained veterinarians. Although the cavalry was of diminishing importance towards the end of the eighteenth century, military dependence on horses for the artillery and for the provision of auxiliary services increased. The effective exploitation of horsepower provided a good solution to the logistical problems involved in contemporary military strategy (Fisher ibid.: 48). In the past, privately contracted farriers had been employed to service the British army's equine needs. However, the changing military use of horses had created problems that such farriers were unable to solve. Using increasingly large numbers of horses to support the artillery involved the concentration of large numbers of animals in single locations for long periods of time. And, if one recalls the ideal conditions for the transmission of infectious disease discussed earlier in this book, such circumstances rendered these horses increasingly vulnerable to contagion. The army thus began to suffer heavy horse losses in times of peace as well as those of war (Fisher ibid.). Glanders, in particular, posed an especial threat during this period, not only to horses, but also to the people who came into contact with them occupationally.[1]

By the close of the eighteenth century, the British army had decided that they should invest in the services of medically educated veterinary professionals, rather than continuing to rely on the traditional cavalry farriers. This decision proved highly fruitful for the military for it resulted in the reduction of horse losses. On the advice of Edward Coleman, a human surgeon who, while lacking veterinary qualifications, had after St Bel's death been appointed to run the London College, the hygiene and ventilation of army stables were greatly improved. Sick animals were isolated or slaughtered, properly buried, and stables were adequately disinfected. The hygienic regime that Coleman suggested to the army was effective, though it should be noted that Coleman himself had no clear knowledge of glanders and its transmission. As a consequence of such advice, the London Veterinary College initially received generous army subsidies that helped secure its future and provided the stimulus for the recruitment of new students who now had the hope of gaining future employment with the military. Military recognition had important repercussions for this fledgling profession for when, in 1805, graduate veterinary surgeons were taken on by the army, they were given the status of commissioned officers. The profession was thus afforded a much greater degree of prestige and although army veterinary surgeons were paid and ranked lower than other army medical professionals, they were now clearly distinct from and had a higher social status than the other people who looked after animals (Fisher ibid.: 49).

When Britain went to war with France in 1793, the need for trained veterinarians to look after the military's horses increased greatly on both sides of the Channel. Coleman's response to this crisis – and to ameliorate the college's finances – was to shorten the length of study, cutting it from the three years that his predecessor St Bel had intended to a mere six months. This was wholly inadequate in comparison to its other European counterparts where veterinary courses had a minimum duration of two years. Even after the war had ended, the length of the London course remained unchanged (Wilkinson 1992: 97). Moreover, Coleman, in his nearly fifty-year reign over the London Veterinary College, later went on to lower the educational standards still further by reducing both fee and entry requirements to increase the numbers of graduates. By 1816, the course had become even shorter (Fisher 1995: 50). Coleman was, by all accounts, a rather arrogant man who firmly believed that animal medicine was not only inferior to human medicine, but also that 'the horse was the only species of domestic animal worthy of any attention at all' (Wilkinson ibid.). Only after Coleman's death in 1839 could the winds of change blow throughout the London Veterinary College and could British veterinary education be brought in line with the higher academic standards and breadth of curriculum that prevailed in the schools of mainland Europe. To this end, a chair of cattle pathology was created in 1842, thus permitting the teaching of the diseases of these economically important domestic animals (Wilkinson ibid.: 102–3). This position was to be filled by James Beart Simonds, a veterinarian who had good practical experience of dealing with cattle disease (Pattison 1990). It was indeed a propitious moment to turn British veterinary attention to the diseases of livestock, for the profession was soon to be put to the test by the resurgence of old, and the coming of new, cattle plagues.

Even into the mid-nineteenth century, the effectiveness and competence of this new-born veterinary profession in dealing with and combating animal disease was still questionable. One of the chief aims of the new veterinary schools had been to put an end to 'quackery' and the 'dangerous practice of farriery' which involved the 'daily sacrificing [of] horses, by mangling the organised parts of the body, without knowing anything of its structure' (Pugh 1962: 72). Veterinary students were to acquire proper knowledge of animal anatomy and physiology. Moreover, the schools that taught them were to establish a distance between the educated veterinary surgeon and the 'barbarous' empirics and farriers that they were intended to usurp. As Roy Porter has pointed out, the veterinary schools would be elegant, enlightened and urban. Human physicians would serve as their 'midwives' in order to 'elevate the new-born veterinary profession above the vulgarity of gelders and blacksmiths' (Porter 1993: 28–9). However, it seems that the early graduates learned little more than the remedies and techniques that were already employed by the more competent farriers of the time. For all their scientific knowledge of animal physiology, the nature of disease and the necessity for good hygiene, the treatments they used 'for most ailments and injuries were as brutally painful as any traditional remedy' (Fisher 1995: 47). Their skills, therefore, were not necessarily more competent or marketable than those of old-style animal doctors that they were meant to replace (Fisher 1993: 296). Furthermore, as we shall shortly see, until the breakthrough of bacteriology in the 1860s and 1870s, in spite of all their 'scientific' education, veterinarians would be as powerless as their lay counterparts in providing therapeutic solutions for the terrible scourges that afflicted European livestock populations (Offringa 1983: 427).

More importantly, well into the nineteenth century, livestock owners continued to demonstrate a great reluctance to exploit the services of these qualified veterinary professionals, instead preferring to continue using the skills of the cow-leeches and blacksmiths to treat the ills and injuries of their animals (Fisher 1995: 47). Although governments legitimised the skills of the educated veterinarian, the farmers continued to rely on the skills of the empirics. In other corners of Europe, empirics steadfastly continued to practise their craft while there was still a market for it. Indeed, as Alexander Numan, physician and principal of the

Rijksveeartsenijschool (Dutch State Veterinary School), observed in 1832, many of those entering the veterinary school came from towns and cities and were completely unfamiliar with the enterprise of farming (Offringa 1983: 424–5). Such a cleft between animal doctor and farmer client undoubtedly did little to foster enthusiasm amongst livestock owners to employ these scientifically trained veterinarians. Competition between these unqualified lay animal healers and qualified veterinary surgeons would indeed continue until the veterinary profession asserted itself and took matters into their own hands in order to protect both their own and the public's interests.[2]

The impact of epizootics in the industrial age

From the late eighteenth century onwards, western Europe underwent a massive growth in population and consequently in animal food demands. The local and national agriculture was often unable to cope with the ever-increasing food demands of the rapidly expanding population. Rather than attempting to intensify domestic food production, the solution to this problem was to supplement existing livestock populations by importing and introducing stock from distant and more thinly populated lands where food-producing animals were cheap and abundant. The technological developments of the industrial age made animal transportation a viable option. The railways and steamships of the nineteenth century were capable of ferrying valuable large animals from one place to another, thus making it possible for foreign livestock to supplement domestic produce. The movement of animals across borders, however, created serious problems for the nations that received the imported livestock.

The repercussions of increased population pressure and the resulting animal importation are exemplified by the situation in the United Kingdom during this era. Until the industrial age, the natural sea boundaries of the British Isles had largely protected their inhabitants – both human and animal – from contagion from abroad. Before animal importation became widespread, serious disease outbreaks amongst livestock populations were fairly sporadic and localised. Moreover, the majority of diseases were indigenous in nature, due to local causes which could in the long term be prevented by improved farm conditions, better nutrition and so forth. Although individual farmers and communities may have experienced great losses, outbreaks could be locally contained through the isolation and slaughter of affected animals. The common practice was to bury the carcasses of animals that had been stricken by disease, so that tainted animal flesh would not end up as human food. This situation changed quite radically as domestic animal food production failed to satisfy the expanding population's growing clamour for cheap and reliable foods of animal origin. The supplementation of domestic livestock with foreign imports to meet these demands, however, brought with it the importation of contagious disease.

Importation was not an entirely new solution to the problem of satisfying the population's food demands. During the eighteenth century, foreign cattle had been imported into Great Britain and had inflicted serious outbreaks of cattle plague on the nation. Mass slaughter and a series of import bans resulted in the eradication of rinderpest from British soil. Strict veterinary control in eastern Europe – from whence the disease originally came – prevented infection from spreading to the west. On the basis of this control, the import embargoes were eventually lifted during the mid-nineteenth century and the trade in live animals was revitalised, the ravages of cattle plague having been pushed to the back of the collective memory (MAFF 1965: 125; Worboys 1992: 54). The reintroduction of rinderpest from mainland Europe – in addition to the introduction of new, highly infectious livestock scourges such as foot-and-mouth disease (first recorded in 1839) and bovine pleuropneumonia (introduced to Britain from pedigree Dutch cattle in 1840) – hit domestic livestock populations hard, resulting in massive losses for livestock holders. Disease spread fast: native animals were exposed to their imported counterparts in markets and shared the same pastures; they travelled across the length and breadth of the country on the roads, by rail or along the waterways, and their flesh was handled by butchers and their carcasses mingled with the domestic product in slaughterhouses and store rooms. Within a relatively short space of time, stock far removed from the original carriers of disease had been exposed to infection (cf. Gamgee 1863, 1866; Fleming 1876). Rinderpest had the most devastating effect since it claimed the vast majority of animals that had been infected; pleuropneumonia had a relatively high mortality rate, and the animals which developed and survived the clinical disease were debilitated by it; foot-and-mouth disease, a highly contagious disease, though not usually a fatal one, resulted in a massive loss of productivity from stock infected by it. The importation of foreign sheep was responsible for the introduction of sheep-pox into Great Britain during the 1840s, which resulted in high mortality and heavy losses for sheep farmers (MAFF 1965: 162–4).

The scarcity of animal food and the desire to stay afloat motivated farmers to dispose of the victims of diseases in a fashion quite different to the traditional practice of burial. A shadowy business steadily grew which offered farmers a far greater return for diseased cattle than the paltry sum that they would receive for the dead animal's hide. Diseased livestock began to be sold and slaughtered for food, since this was more profitable than attempting to cure them from their affliction. As John Gamgee, perhaps the most vocal veterinarian of the time, lamented, it was now the farmer's practice to 'generate disease and sell diseased stock', rather than to seek any veterinary attention or treatment for affected animals (Gamgee 1863: 6). The trade in diseased livestock was certainly an unhealthy one, for both the animals and the public at large. The quality of meat fell, while the price of it soared; contaminated and unattractive carcasses were dressed up by butchers to make them more attractive to unwitting consumers both rich and poor.

During the 1850s, impressed by the standards of veterinary medicine in mainland Europe and incensed by the British government's failure to appreciate the need for animal disease control, Gamgee began to campaign vigorously for government reform in Britain and the (international) control of infectious animal disease. He was a strict proponent of the notion of contagionism, believing that epizootic diseases could only ever spread through contact and would do so under any given conditions. This was in contrast to the anti-contagionists who held that 'such diseases might in fact arise spontaneously, erupting whenever and wherever conditions were favourable' (Worboys 1992: 54). As an ardent champion of germ theory, Gamgee set about trying to convince both the British government and the veterinary medical establishment that they should adopt new measures to prevent the potential devastation that future livestock disease might bring in its wake. In a report to the Privy Council in 1862, Gamgee proposed that drastic changes be made in the cattle trade and that special markets to process foreign stock and a state veterinary inspectorate be established. In his view, the existing free trade in cattle was equatable to a free trade in cattle disease. However, although the importation and trade in livestock had posed clear dangers with regard to disease, outbreaks of both foot-and-mouth disease and pleuropneumonia, while undesirable, had not produced spectacular losses in livestock numbers and income (MAFF 1965: 126). Even the livestock farmers who were the most directly affected by such outbreaks tended to regard animal disease as an occupational hazard (Fisher 1979/80: 49). Largely for this reason, Gamgee's words fell on deaf ears, but his public warnings of the dangers of importation and disease were prophetic of the devastation that was to come. The following year, Gamgee played a key role in convening the very first European veterinary congress in Hamburg to discuss the international problems created by epizootic disease. Delegates came mainly from Prussia, Austria and Switzerland and divulged their own broad practical experiences in dealing with animal disease in their own countries (Gamgee 1866). Again, the damning evidence – of the inadequacies of disease control and livestock regulations in Britain, in comparison with its European counterparts – that this congress produced was ignored by the British authorities. Likewise, the portentous letters published in *The Times*, that Gamgee addressed to Sir George Grey and other members of the Privy Council, went unheeded. For example, in seeking trade restrictions, Gamgee implored that

> I am not dealing with imaginary evils when I have before my eyes as I write this letter a statement of the losses sustained by the Russian Plague in the Austrian dominions. During the past fourteen years, 500,000 animals have been seized by the disease, and of these 270,000 died. Even that loss is comparatively small when contrasted with the loss we have sustained during the last eighteen or twenty years through the lung disease; but if Russian cattle manage to reach our markets – and why should they not? – we shall certainly have more than the Austrians, whose organisation for the prevention of disease amongst cattle is perhaps the best in Europe. Prudent men must agree with me, that under existing circumstances we need something more than the rapid transmission of stock from foreign to British markets. We have already too much occasion to lament the introduction of foreign diseases into these islands, and we must watch lest we henceforth find that, whereas wheat barely remunerates the tiller of the soil for his labour, disease among livestock may irretrievably ruin him.
>
> (MAFF 1965: 14)

It was only in 1865, when an outbreak of rinderpest – of the kind feared greatly by John Gamgee – decimated British livestock, that the government realised that they required an effective body of specialists to be able to deal with the great threat to the economy and public posed by animal disease. Finally, the Privy Council conceded and established a Veterinary Department to deal with the cattle plague that same year. This move marks the inception of an organised state veterinary service in Britain (MAFF 1965: 125–7).

The outbreak of cattle plague of 1865 was a devastating one. It was traced to a shipment of oxen and sheep that had arrived in Britain on 29 May 1865 from eastern Europe. Some of these cattle turned out to be diseased, though they had passed the port inspectors in Hull and been sent to London and Manchester; the first reports of disease came from a London dairy (ibid.: 127–8). From then on, the disease raged throughout Britain killing cattle by their thousands and threatening farmers with ruin. By the following year, several efforts at parliamentary reform had been made in a bid to prevent future calamities. Gamgee continued to highlight the importance of regulating and controlling cattle livestock. He believed that movement of livestock should cease from wherever the cattle plague had appeared and that importation from the Netherlands should be prohibited since many outbreaks could be traced back to shipments from Dutch ports. Further to this, Gamgee advocated a system of national insurance or indemnity to compensate farmers for their losses, in addition to the slaughter of all sick and infected animals (Gamgee 1866: vi). More importantly, he was against any attempts to treat the plague through vaccination as had been proposed by others. Eradication through slaughter and a stop on animal traffic was, he argued, the only rational solution (ibid.: viii–ix).

Even after events had proved his point, Gamgee's proposals still continued to meet resistance, and public attempts were made to ridicule him. Contagionism, in particular, came under attack. Thus, Strickland Constable, one of Gamgee's most caustic opponents and a man highly sceptical about theories of contagion, wrote copiously on Gamgee's 'veterinary delusions'. In a letter to a Yorkshire newspaper, he declared that

> We profess not to believe in witchcraft now, but our credulity and superstitions only happen to take other forms. A great many years ago, when the black death raged, people in their ignorance and credulity, believed, from

> consulting their imaginations instead of facts, that wells were poisoned by the Jews; and the Jews were slaughtered accordingly. Now we are all believing, in the same way, by consulting our imaginations instead of facts, that infection is carried by the winds, and by birds and dogs, and we are slaughtering our cattle accordingly, where is the difference in the degree of superstition between these two cases . . . The truth is, all we can say, with reason and without superstition, is that facts show that one beast will often, but not certainly, catch the disease directly from another, but that there are no facts whatever to warrant belief in any further degree either of infection or contagion.
>
> (Strickland Constable 1866: 98–9)

The 'butcher's knife', he concluded, was the 'real rinderpest, for that was incurable' (Strickland Constable 1866: 29).[3] The veterinary profession in general was at this time increasingly blamed for its inability to protect Britain from the disease (Worboys 1992: 55). As one commentator, declining to be named in full, wrote, 'when you send for the veterinary surgeon, order a grave to be dug, and prepare to pay a long bill' ('E.H.' 1865: 3). There were, however, voices of reason that provided more practical advice to farmers in preventing the spread of the dreaded rinderpest. For example, a Scottish tenant farmer, also choosing to remain anonymous, counselled his readers on the necessity of isolating everything from an infected locality. Buried dead cattle, he advised, should be quick-limed; straw, manure and refuse burnt with tar and brushwood; utensils and farm equipment disinfected with permanganate of potash, as should all persons who had come into contact with the animals, and their clothing should be burned. Complete isolation, he argued, should be unremittingly enforced for 'it is useless otherwise to kill the animals; the infection will be left for the newcomers, and all that is done in the slaughtering will be lost' ('Scottish Tenant Farmer' 1866: 14).

Throughout late 1865 and 1866, public opinion was still divided and the Royal Commission, which had been appointed to investigate cattle plague, failed to come up with a good solution to the management of animal disease. Only when the situation worsened were the drastic measures advised by John Gamgee actually adopted and entered into the statute books under the guise of the Cattle Diseases Prevention Bill. By September 1867, the success of these measures became evident and rinderpest was eradicated from Great

Britain (MAFF 1965: 130–4). Similar measures were applied in the future and a series of new legislative attempts, such as The Contagious Diseases (Animals) Act and Animals Order, were made and adapted from 1876 onwards in order to contain other infectious animal diseases. In the meantime, the losses to rinderpest suffered by British farmers, since its initial outbreak in 1865, had been estimated at 420,000 cattle out of a population of around 6,000,000. This meant a national average of seven per cent, though in the most severely affected areas, such as Cheshire, losses were estimated at around 50 to 66 per cent (MAFF 1965: 134).

Although the effects of cattle plague were severe and fervently debated, the subject did not really touch the hearts and minds of the masses, illustrating the extent to which livestock disease truly affected the majority of people in this new industrial age. While rinderpest and its control received media attention – numerous letters and cartoons parodying the chief protagonists in the parliamentary debate having been published in national newspapers – active discussion and outcry was generally limited to a fairly small number of people. It was really only farmers, veterinarians, medical specialists and people involved in the live animal trade who actually participated in the debate about the spread and containment of cattle plague. Public interest and outcry was rather transitory and, when the worst was over, the devastation that rinderpest left behind was largely forgotten. The urban population simply did not have to pick up the pieces that cattle plague left in its wake. They were in fact more concerned with the stray and neglected dogs which roamed the streets and posed a more visible threat to their own well-being in the – often imagined – form of a much rarer disease: rabies (Ritvo 1987a; Swabe 1995).

On mainland Europe, outbreaks of rinderpest played considerable havoc with livestock populations and the agricultural economy. In France, where the action against the disease had been well coordinated and preventative regulations had been ruthlessly enforced, losses were successfully minimised. However, in the Netherlands, like Britain, where the fight against the cattle plague was improperly coordinated, the epizootic resulted in great mortality amongst cattle and considerable economic damage (Fisher 1993: 301). Although the Dutch government had begun to concern itself with the effects of infectious cattle diseases back in the 1840s, the legislation that it instituted proved ineffective with the arrival of a fresh scourge of rinderpest in 1865. In May 1840 and July 1842, two Acts had been passed with a view to managing a special

Agricultural Fund, contributed to by farmers, that would compensate them for their losses sustained during serious outbreaks of livestock disease. Licensed empirics and trained veterinary surgeons from the State Veterinary School in Utrecht were appointed in order to decide whether compensation should be paid and diseased animals sent to slaughter. The failure to report infectious cattle disease or isolate sick animals, in addition to infecting other people's cattle, was made a punishable offence by the 1840 Act. The revised version added further charges to this list (Kerstens 1971: 15–16). However, by 1849, after repeated outbreaks of pleuropneumonia, the Agricultural Fund had dried up completely. This, Offringa (1983) suggests, had the interesting side-effect of going some way in enhancing the rather uncomfortable relationship between farmers and veterinarians. For whereas previously it had been the veterinary surgeon who deemed whether animals should be destroyed, making him a most unwelcome visitor on farms, it was now no longer possible to slaughter animals for financial compensation; the veterinarian therefore became a desirable cohort. After all, the veterinarians could diagnose an animal's complaint and the farmer could decide for himself whether he would get rid of the animal – often by sale to another unwitting farmer. This, Offringa argues, heralded a new complicity between farmers and veterinarians (Offringa 1983: 427–8).

The exhaustion of the communal fund led in turn to the institution of a Compulsory Purchase Act in 1851, which instead made public funds available to back the fight against contagious livestock disease. In addition to this, a further act was passed in October 1865 that made it possible to institute measures to control the import and movement of cattle from abroad and to prohibit cattle markets from being held. This act also imposed regulations on the notification of contagious disease, the sale, treatment and inspection of cattle – live or dead – meat, animal hides, wool, manure and so forth. It was necessary to introduce this new act, because it appeared that rinderpest had been reintroduced into the Netherlands by unsold cattle that had been re-imported from Britain without adequate control (Kerstens 1971: 16). It was thus in July 1865 that rinderpest returned with a vengeance to afflict Dutch cattle (Offringa 1971: 111). In order to combat this new threat to the agricultural economy, G.J. Hengeveld, a professor from the veterinary school and supporter of the contagion theory, was called in to conduct research on the disease and to make scientific recommendations for its control and eradication to the government; a commission of veterinary surgeons was established in order to advise ministers on the crisis. They recommended that the following measures should be taken: infected areas should be sealed off with a double military cordon; all diseased or suspect cattle in infected areas should be seized and slaughtered; import and transit traffic should cease along the country's frontiers, including the seizure and destruction of all infected railway cattle wagons; cattle markets should be prohibited throughout the land; and, finally, local authorities should issue appropriate by-laws and be afforded the necessary veterinary assistance, financial support and policing (Kerstens 1971: 16).

It turned out to be constitutionally impossible to act on all of these recommendations. An act incorporating the remaining prohibitions was passed in October 1865, but was then revoked when it was discovered that local authorities were ignoring or being negligent in utilising their powers to control the spread of infection (Kerstens 1971: 16). Moreover, it seems that Thorbecke, the liberal prime minister of the day, was far from keen on such recommendations and did not wish to intervene too rigorously. He contended that it would be too expensive for the state to pay for the destruction of animals suspected of harbouring or having the disease. Moreover, he saw the prevention of livestock disease primarily as the task of local councils and provincial authorities. This approach proved disastrous and it was only in 1867 when Thorbecke had been replaced by Heemskerk, a rather more conservative politician, that the epizootic was contained through the institution of an effective slaughter policy (Offringa 1983: 428). The farmers were largely responsible for the failure of these well-intentioned efforts to eradicate the cattle plague, for they refused to willingly succumb to the new regulations regarding livestock seizure, destruction, disposal and disinfection. Before such measures could be carried out, military force had to be employed to convince Dutch farmers to obey the letter of the law. A number of farmers were killed while resisting these measures, before the rest submitted and grudgingly agreed to have their livestock expropriated (Kerstens 1971: 19). In some cases, particularly in the provinces of South Holland and Utrecht, farmers refused to have their animals destroyed on religious grounds. These areas were also the worst hit. By the time the crisis had come to an end, the economic damage and extent of livestock losses were colossal. From the initial outbreak in July 1865 to its eventual eradication in December 1867, 156,711 cattle had been affected; of this number, 78,133 died of the disease, 27,021 were destroyed and 51,565 recovered. The economic damage was estimated at a grand total of 13 million guilders (Offringa 1971: 113).

As in Britain, the devastation of this major rinderpest epizootic provided the impetus for the establishment of a state veterinary service in the Netherlands. In 1868, a bill was drafted and submitted to the States-General, which would lay the groundwork for the establishment of a system of government inspection of livestock health. After lengthy discussions, a new version of this bill was accepted and received royal assent in July 1870. By December 1870, a royal decree had been issued that clearly set out which animal diseases should be deemed contagious, and the measures and methods that the state should take in order to eradicate and control future outbreaks. The following diseases were designated as contagious livestock diseases: rinderpest in ruminants; pleuropneumonia in cattle; malignant foot-and-mouth disease in cattle and sheep; glanders in equines; scabies in horses and sheep; sheep-pox; anthrax; and rabies in all livestock. In January 1871, the Dutch Veterinary Service came into being, with a number of state-appointed district veterinary surgeons and their deputies employed to carry out inspections and to enforce new regulations pertaining to the management of animal diseases (Kerstens 1971: 19–22; I.J.R.Visser 1996). The institution of the Veterinary Service thus provided important new employment opportunities for graduate veterinarians, outside of private practice or the military (Offringa 1983: 428). The new measures proved effective and, after the institution of a new act in 1878 that laid down new powers for the control of pleuropneumonia in specific parts of the Netherlands, this serious cattle disease that had raged in the country on and off since 1831 was finally eradicated after an effective campaign in 1887. Sheep-pox also made its last appearance in 1893 (Kerstens 1971: 22).

Intensifying the veterinary regime

The great cattle plague of 1865 thus highlighted the inefficacy of the existing veterinary regime and the necessity of effective state intervention and control. In many respects, this epizootic can be regarded as a critical episode in the development of organised and state-directed animal disease control, much in the same way as the nineteenth-century cholera epidemics discussed by Abram de Swaan (1988) can be perceived as a critical occurrence in the development of state-regulated public health and hygiene measures. In addition to this, the rinderpest epizootic of 1865 illustrated that the problem of animal disease – and consequently animal disease control – could not be confined within the bounds of individual nations. Disease organisms do not recognise international borders, and the increasing traffic of both livestock and animal carcasses between nations that the developments of the late eighteenth and nineteenth centuries brought in their wake created the ideal circumstances for increased opportunities for disease transmission. This inadequate hygiene and a lack of regulation and control added up to a real recipe for disaster. The growing complexity of the web of interdependencies between individuals, both human and animal, during this period had thus created a situation where infectious animal disease could gain a stranglehold on both the livestock population and the human agricultural economy.

The emerging globalisation of animal disease problems can be well illustrated by events surrounding the rinderpest epizootic of 1865. Infected livestock, moved by sea from eastern Europe to and then through Britain and then on to the Netherlands, allowed the disease-causing organisms to travel with considerable ease, finding new and vulnerable hosts as they went. European governments imposed their own measures – with differing degrees of efficiency – to curtail the spread of the disease and limit both livestock losses and economic damage. However, it became clear that the problem at hand was of international importance. Further International Veterinary Congresses, one in Vienna in 1865 and another in Zürich in 1867, were held in an attempt to draw up international regulations to control and eradicate the cattle plague. Delegates attended from Austria, Hungary, Belgium, France, Germany, Great Britain, Italy, Rumania, Russia, Switzerland, Serbia and Turkey; the Dutch were notably absent at the Vienna meeting but agreed with the main conclusion of the congress, i.e. rapid international communication in the event of outbreaks of cattle plague (MAFF 1965: 39–40). Such early attempts to internationalise livestock importation regulations and animal disease control provide a precursor to the latter bids to internationalise and consolidate the veterinary regime that will be discussed in the following chapter.

While this great crisis had been going on in European agriculture, the original problem – namely increasing demands for animal produce – that had precipitated the importation of foreign livestock to supplement the domestic product remained unsolved. The population of western European nations continued to expand as economic prosperity increased due to the success and growth of the new manufacturing industries. Again, this problem can be illustrated by the situation in Britain, which was still the most advanced industrial nation in Europe. Although the importation of foreign stock had initially provided a quick and easy solution to this problem, the disease that it had brought with it left people looking for new answers to satisfy consumer demands. The key to solving this problem lay many thousands of miles away in Britain's distant colonies of Australia and New Zealand, where cattle and sheep could be found in over-abundance. In Australia, a major new trade began by exploiting these untapped animal resources by slaughtering them, tinning and then exporting their meat to Britain. During the first year of this trade in 1867, 286,526 pounds of tinned beef had been shipped from one side of the world to the other; by 1880, the total had reached some 16 million (MAFF 1965: 46). There was also a glut of cattle in North America and from the 1870s, live cattle were increasingly exported to Britain, although mortality during the long sea voyage added extra costs to the meat. Experiments with refrigeration techniques eventually provided an answer to this problem and in 1877 the first cargo of 'chilled' beef was shipped from New York to Britain. With this new international meat trade, it became a possibility for the trade in live food animals to be stopped and for the native livestock population to properly recover from the battering it had taken from earlier epidemics. It was thought, even by John Gamgee who by that time had ceased practising veterinary medicine in favour of experimenting with refrigeration, that the importation of chilled meat would be unlikely to result in the introduction of foreign animal diseases: as it turns out, he was wrong (MAFF 1965: 47).

While the great cattle plague of 1865 highlighted the inadequacies of existing measures for animal disease control, it also emphasised the necessity of both improving veterinary education and raising the public's confidence in the profession. During the course of the epizootic in Britain, it had become increasingly evident that qualified veterinary surgeons were quite ignorant not only of the cattle plague, but also of the diseases of cattle in general. Veterinarians increasingly came under fire from farmers who criticised their incompetence in diagnosing or misdiagnosing rinderpest and their lack of adequate action in dealing with the disease. Their veterinary education failed to provide them with the means and knowledge to fight against infectious cattle disease. In spite of Simonds' professorship in cattle pathology at the Royal Veterinary College, London, it was still possible for students to qualify as fully-fledged veterinary surgeons without having acquired any practical knowledge of livestock disease. It is then no wonder that farmers were disinclined to let veterinary surgeons anywhere near their cattle, preferring instead the lay attentions of the cow-leech who at least had practical experience in dealing with these animals (Fisher 1993: 285–7). In the Netherlands, too, farmers remained somewhat sceptical about the proficiency and competence of these scientifically educated veterinarians in treating their livestock (Offringa 1983).

Moreover, at this time, the veterinary profession had yet to attain a fully professional status; in Britain, for example, veterinarians were ranked far below human medical practitioners and, despite their formal training, were, as a profession, generally classified at the same level as the farriers and cow-leeches whom they despised. They therefore needed to formally differentiate themselves from such people in order to advance their social standing. To this end, a Veterinary Surgeons Bill was put forward in 1866 by the Royal College of Veterinary Surgeons, but was soon to be abandoned due to the apparent failings of the profession and its standards of education that had been highlighted by the disastrous events surrounding the cattle plague. The aim of this bill had been to improve the income, social status and standards of professional competence of veterinarians; largely with a view to restricting the competition from the multifarious and unqualified animal doctors who continued to step into the formally educated veterinarians' shoes, often at the animal owner's behest. Although a royal charter to protect the veterinary profession from these uneducated men had been established in 1844, the unqualified could still call themselves veterinary surgeons and impede the qualified veterinary surgeon in his attempts to earn a decent income (Fisher 1993: 287–8). Reform in veterinary education was thus necessary if the veterinary profession was to gain statutory recognition and to attain the monopoly on treating animals in health and disease. The personal and institutional rivalries that were rife between existing veterinary schools would have to come to an end, as would the predominant role of medical, rather than veterinary surgeons in veterinary training. The entry requirements for study would also have to be raised considerably, including both basic literacy and numeracy skills. Moreover, the curriculum would have to be extended to adequately encompass livestock and their diseases (Fisher ibid.: 290–2).

It was the eventual establishment of the Veterinary Department of the Privy Council in response to the cattle plague of 1865 that laid the groundwork for the future success of the British veterinary profession. The new legislation that was created to deal with the problems of animal disease control created new opportunities for veterinarians to be employed in an official governmental capacity. Veterinarians were not only employed directly by the department as inspectors, but local authorities were also obliged to appoint qualified veterinary surgeons; thereby guaranteeing the qualified a monopoly over the provision of veterinary services in the public sector. An almost identical development occurred concurrently in the Netherlands with the establishment of the State Veterinary Service, for the employment of veterinarians by the state also permitted the social consolidation of the profession (cf. Offringa 1983). By 1881, the Royal College of Veterinary Surgeons succeeded, through legislation, to improve the lot of their profession in the same manner that had been attempted in 1866. The veterinary colleges managed to get their act together and greatly raised entrance standards and diversified the nature of the curriculum. As the twentieth century approached, the level of competence of qualified veterinarians began to show signs of definite improvement (Fisher 1993: 300–1).

Likewise, in the Netherlands, legislation instituted in 1874 pertaining to the practice of veterinary medicine set down clear criteria for both qualified veterinarians and existing empirics. In order to continue practising their art, empirics were now obliged to pass a special examination – new ones were no longer tolerated. Similarly, veterinary education was to be afforded a much higher academic status. Following the example of a number of prominent veterinary schools in Germany that had been raised to the level of *Tierärtzliche Hochschulen* between 1888 and 1890, in 1896 the Dutch Society for the Improvement of Veterinary Medicine and Livestock Breeding – established some fourteen years previously – demanded that the State Veterinary School be accorded the status of an institute of higher learning also. Accompanying this move came a plea to scrap the existing admission exam and to accept new students on the basis of their final secondary school diplomas, thus raising the general educational standards of pupils and consequently the overall prestige of the institution also. By 1904, the possession of these diplomas had become the standard for entrance to the veterinary school and, by 1925, the school had officially been incorporated into the structure of the State University of Utrecht (Offringa 1976: 168). In Germany, some of the veterinary schools had already had university connections since they had been established and all had attained the rank of academies by 1887. Passing a university admission examination to gain entrance to a veterinary school had been in place in Bavaria since 1851, followed by Bern in 1870, Zurich in 1878 and France in 1881. This too marks the increasingly academic nature and rising status of the veterinary profession in Europe during the second half of the nineteenth century (Ackerknecht and Fischer-Homberger 1977: 261).

Microbiological breakthrough

A major factor in the legitimisation of the veterinary profession was the important medical scientific breakthroughs that took place during the second half of the nineteenth century. In particular, the development of bacteriology was to have far-reaching consequences for the veterinary regime and its efficacy. The discovery of pathogenic bacteria revolutionised veterinary medical science for it finally provided veterinarians with the scientific tools with which they could both prevent and employ therapeutic measures in the fight against animal disease (Offringa 1983). Bacteria had in fact first been observed under the microscope of the Dutch naturalist Antonie van Leeuwenhoek back in the late seventeenth century (Wilkinson 1992: 30). However, it was to take some two hundred years before the science of bacteriology was to develop and the belief that bacteria were spontaneously generated, which dominated medical science, would gradually be supplanted by the notion of germ theory that had been fiercely debated throughout the mid-nineteenth century. The idea that disease was spread through contagion had been conjectured for many years, but was only to be corroborated in the latter half of the nineteenth century by a variety of experimental studies, the most famous of which were conducted by the French chemist and biologist Louis Pasteur during the 1860s and the German scientist Robert Koch in the 1870s.

Pasteur's work on the process of fermentation in alcohol and milk eventually led him to conclude that disease could be caused by microscopic organisms. Pasteur had been able to demonstrate, as had been thought by other scientists previously, that yeast played a clear role in the process of fermentation. More importantly, he showed that wine sometimes became sour due to the presence of additional organisms such as bacteria. These bacteria, he advised, could be eliminated through heat treatment. Later, he extended his investigations to the souring of milk and applied an identical solution to the problem by heating milk to 65°C for thirty minutes before bottling it, thus preventing it from going sour and killing infectious agents. This process became known as pasteurisation and has been a crucial factor in maintaining veterinary public health since its widespread introduction in milk production. Pasteur saw a clear analogy between the development of disease and the process of fermentation. In the same way that undesirable microorganisms invade alcohol or milk causing it to sour, disease, he postulated, arose when germs attacked the human or animal body from the outside. In 1865, Pasteur began experiments on silkworms, in a bid to understand the nature of a disease that was seriously disrupting the French silk industry. His investigations revealed that the microscopic matter that could be found in diseased silkworms, moths and eggs were actually disease-producing organisms. On this basis, he developed a method of control that involved the selection of disease-free eggs for silk production and which ultimately saved the silk industry from catastrophe. Pasteur then turned his attention to the nature and causes of animal disease, singling out fowl cholera and anthrax as his first subjects of study (Dunlop and Williams 1996: 380–3).

Around the same time, Koch – quite independently of his French contemporary – began investigating the causes of anthrax. It had already been established in 1856, by Koch's fellow countryman and veterinarian Frederick Brauell who had managed to transmit the disease from people to sheep, that anthrax was indeed a zoonotic disease. Likewise, in 1860, Henri Mamer Onésime Delafond, the director of the Alfort veterinary school and a previous exponent of humoral pathology, described the rod-shaped bodies that he – and others before him – had observed in the blood of anthrax-infected animals and went on to cultivate them *in vitro*, speculating that these were the cause of the disease (Wilkinson 1992: 128). Koch continued in the spirit of Brauell's research, but instead decided to tackle the problem – as Delafond had done fifteen years earlier – of culturing the organism that he thought caused the disease *in vitro*. He developed a novel system of culture plates, using first potato slices, then meat extract solidified with gelatine and later with agar as a nutrient medium, and involving special small glass dishes invented by his assistant, Richard Petri. This technique proved highly successful and in 1877 Koch was eventually able to isolate the anthrax bacillus, proving that anthrax was caused by a specific microorganism (Brock 1961: 89–95). The repercussions of this discovery were enormous, for it was the very first time that it had been demonstrated, beyond reasonable doubt, that a single causative agent was responsible for a disease. Koch also paved the way for contemporary and future researchers for he provided an example of how one should work with microorganisms, how they should be extracted from infected animals, how they could be cultivated artificially and, more importantly, how they could be destroyed. Koch went on to study the bacterial infection of wounds and later to identify the bacillus that caused tuberculosis (Brock 1988: 117–37).

The late 1870s also bore witness to the first attempts to develop vaccines for the prevention of animal diseases. In the field of human medicine, Edward Jenner's cowpox vaccine, which he first tested on a human subject in 1796, had proved invaluable in the fight against smallpox (Brock 1961: 121–5). However, more than seven decades were to pass before Jenner's ideas and technique were to be successfully employed to deal with other diseases. It is particularly notable that animal, rather than human disease provided the inspiration and materials for the development of the first successful vaccines. Perhaps this can be seen as a reflection of the impact of animal disease on late-nineteenth-century society and the necessity of preventing and controlling it. In 1879, Jean-Joseph-Henri Toussaint, a graduate of the Lyon veterinary school, succeeded in the *in vitro* cultivation of the infectious agent responsible for fowl cholera, a disease resulting in mortality in chickens. In turn, Toussaint furnished Louis Pasteur with a sample of this culture, providing Pasteur with the basis for the initial development of his very first vaccine that same year. Although Toussaint was responsible for cultivating the organism that caused fowl cholera, it was instead to be named *Pasteurella* in honour of his more famous colleague. The following year, Toussaint began experimenting with the possibilities of rendering sheep resistant to anthrax infection. Again, Pasteur was quick to follow and in 1881 he applied the technique, that he had developed previously for vaccination against fowl cholera, to anthrax. Pasteur had found that by cultivating *Bacillus anthracis* at a temperature of 42°C to 43°C, it lost its virulence. When animals were vaccinated with these attenuated bacilli, they displayed immunity when exposure to the disease should have been fatal. Pasteur went on to study the causes and prevention by means of vaccination of a whole host of other diseases, the most famous of which became the post-exposure prophylaxis he developed against rabies. Though yet again, as Lise Wilkinson observes, Pasteur achieved this success by riding on the back of the work of a much lesser-known scientist. In the case of rabies, it was to be another Lyon graduate, Pierre-Victor Galtier, who first demonstrated that sheep could be protected from rabies through subcutaneous inoculation with the saliva obtained from a rabid dog. Galtier identified the rabbit as being the ideal subject for the study of rabies, which also became Pasteur's chosen experimental species. Galtier's contributions to the prevention of rabies have since been greatly overlooked, Pasteur receiving all the acclaim for the development of an attenuated form of the virus that could be used in the inoculation of humans against the virus which causes this much-feared zoonotic disease (Wilkinson 1992: 154–60).

Such early developments in the science of bacteriology and immunology – and the countless other studies of animal disease and its prevention that were to follow – provided the veterinary profession with the tools with which it could effectively fight against animal disease and win the confidence of their farmer clients. The farming world, for example, clamoured for Pasteur's anthrax vaccine to put an end to this terrible disease that had caused great mortality in livestock, particularly sheep, and impeded wool production for centuries. A further veterinary problem not related directly to bacterial disease, but one that benefited from the increasing acceptance of germ theory, was that of treating wound infection. From the mid-nineteenth century onwards, various physicians had observed the necessity for increased hygiene in order to prevent contamination and thus unnecessary mortality amongst patients. For example, the British surgeon Joseph Lister had concluded that wounds became septic due to the germs that entered them from the air. In 1865, he adopted the measure of spraying his surgery with carbolic acid that would act as an antiseptic to prevent infections occurring, and sterilising surgical equipment in boiling water (Brock 1961: 86–9). The adoption of antiseptic surgery within veterinary practice proved extremely beneficial to the treatment of animals (Dunlop and Williams 1996: 397–8). Although such developments were to revolutionise the practice and effectiveness of veterinary medicine, these new methods and ideas were not taken on board immediately by the veterinary establishment. As Offringa notes of Dutch veterinary education, it was to take a fair while before the old guard who relied on the precepts of humoral pathology for their diagnoses and blood-letting for their therapy were to be replaced by a new generation of veterinary instructors who would bring the profession and its ideas rather more up-to-date (Offringa 1983: 429).

The increasing importance of veterinary public health

From the late nineteenth century onwards, veterinary medical science began to play an increasingly important role in the preservation and protection of public health. Although the term *veterinary public health* was only to be introduced during the latter half of the twentieth century (Schwabe 1984a: 9), it is nonetheless appropriate to describe the involvement of nineteenth-century veterinarians in the control of diseases that affect both animal and humans and the production of animal-derived produce in such terms. As the above discussion has illustrated, the increasing urbanisation of society led to decreasing everyday contact with animals – and consequently exposure to animal disease – for the vast majority of the population. Yet although the ever-growing urban populace of European nations seldom endured the trials and tribulations of agrarian life, they were nevertheless still at risk from the effects of animal disease in their urban lives. Anthrax, for example, was an occupational hazard for those working within the new woollen industry of the nineteenth century. Commonly known as 'woolsorters' disease', it became the scourge of the industry resulting in fatalities amongst workers. In the 1870s, consternation amongst British wool workers grew as the number of deaths increased, in apparent coincidence with the expanding use of wool and hair from eastern Europe. Otherwise able-bodied men died suddenly, leaving behind their dependants who often had to turn to the workhouses to survive. Improved sanitation and the proper disinfection of fleeces before human handling was eventually advised to prevent the infection of workers, but no code of rules was actually adopted by the British wool industry until 1897. After this time, the mortality rate amongst wool workers from anthrax declined significantly (Cunningham 1976: 169–70). Anthrax, however, was not just transmissible through contact with infected fleeces, it was – like several other important zoonotic diseases – communicable to humans through the consumption of infected animal produce.

Illness and death caused by eating foods of animal origin was in fact the greatest animal hazard with which the mid-nineteenth-century urban populations of Europe had to contend. It was thus during this period that veterinarians began to play an increasingly important role in protecting human health within the field of meat inspection. As discussed earlier, an extremely unhealthy trade in selling the flesh of diseased livestock had grown up in Britain during the nineteenth century leading to a decline in the quality of meat on sale to the consumer. Few explicit references to the inspection of meat can actually be found in British legislation until 1875, when a Public Health Act was instituted that permitted the seizure of unsound meat and diseased animals by designated medical health officers and sanitary inspectors; this act was to be further amended in 1890 (MAFF 1965: 283). A similar trade in diseased meat could also be found during the nineteenth century in the Netherlands. There too a lucrative business emerged involving not only the sale of meat from slaughtered animals that had been infected with rinderpest, pleuropneumonia, anthrax, tuberculosis, glanders, tapeworms and trichinosis, but also flesh from animals that had simply died. Knackers travelled to farms far and wide to collect cadavers with their dog carts, even digging up rotting carcasses to be brought back to the knacker's yard to be processed into pies and sausages that were fraudulently sold on to and consumed by the public, especially the lower classes (Koolmees 1997: 90–3). This illicit meat trade presented enormous risks to public health and highlighted the necessity of state intervention in meat hygiene control. From the 1850s onwards, after numerous outbreaks of trichinosis and meat poisoning, local authorities began to address the problem of meat hygiene and even attempted to institute a mandatory and centralised system of municipal slaughterhouses where animals would be slaughtered under professional veterinary supervision. However, only three of such public abattoirs were actually to be built during the last quarter of the nineteenth century. It was to be the next century before an adequate meat inspection service and effective legislation were to be established in the Netherlands (Koolmees 1997: 279).

The first calls for state intervention and the necessity of meat inspection had in fact been made many years earlier during the late eighteenth century by a German physician, Johann Peter Frank. Frank, a pioneer of social medicine, had recognised the importance of the quality of the food that people consumed for their state of health and regarded meat inspection as a governmental responsibility. He called for the professional veterinary supervision of slaughterhouse activities and the centralisation of slaughter in proper and hygienic public abattoirs. Frank also identified the need for a proper scientific basis to the practice of meat inspection, which was then greatly lacking. At the time, there was great resistance to Frank's enlightened ideas about public health reforms (Koolmees 1997: 66–7). An organised system of meat inspection, along the lines that Frank suggested, was only set up in Germany after serious outbreaks of trichinosis during the 1860s. Public slaughterhouses and new legislation were established as a consequence of such epidemics. For instance, by 1868 the Prussian authorities required that all animals must be slaughtered in public slaughterhouses under veterinary supervision and inspection (Schwabe 1984a: 539). It was to be in France that such early ideas about public health found more fertile ground. The French Revolution accorded all citizens equal rights to good health and provided new bureaucratic possibilities for state intervention in matters such as the supervision of slaughter and meat inspection (Koolmees 1997: 66–7). However, while the political conditions in France were appropriate to providing the basis for state intervention in matters of veterinary public health, research produced by the French veterinary schools indicated that meat from animals infected with rinderpest posed no threat to human health. Though rinderpest is indeed not a zoonotic disease, such findings were used to back up claims that the meat from animals suffering from other infectious diseases was not harmful to people (Dunlop and Williams 1996: 576).

By the mid-nineteenth century, as demands for meat continued to grow and the trade in diseased meat flourished, a more scientific basis for meat inspection was clearly required. Developments in the field of parasitology during the 1850s were to provide important scientific corroboration of the transmission of animal disease to humans through the consumption of infected meat. For example, in 1855, Friedrich Küchenmeister demonstrated a relationship between a parasite affecting pigs and the tapeworms that afflicted humans. A similar discovery linking a bovine parasite also to the human tapeworm was made by Rudolf Leuckart in 1861. Another parasite significant to the communication of animal disease to humans through the consumption of infected meat was the *Trichinella spiralis*. These roundworms that mainly live in the intestines of rats and pigs were responsible for trichinosis, a serious – and often deadly – infection that can be transmitted to humans through the consumption of raw or improperly cooked meat. Until 1860, this parasite was regarded as harmless. However, after research conducted by Friedrich A. Zenker, Rudolf Virchow and Leuckart, it was discovered that these parasites could indeed be extremely damaging to human health. The aforementioned epidemics of trichinosis in Germany are exemplary of the effects of eating contaminated pig products raw (Koolmees 1997: 99–100). Such advances in parasitology established a scientific basis for the inspection of meat products and aroused increasing interest in the issue of food safety. This combined with the contemporary development of pathogenic bacteriology, as discussed above, which also highlighted the dangers that bacteria in food may pose to human health stimulated this interest still further. For example, J-A. Villemin's discovery in 1865 that tuberculosis could indeed cross the species divide was crucial to instituting new measures to ensure the inspection of both livestock and meat (Offringa 1983: 429).

With such developments at hand, the veterinary profession was able to find another new niche in the market for their services. That is, however, not to say that there was no competition from other medical professionals who regarded the issue of meat inspection as part and parcel of their own professional domain and requiring their expert theoretical knowledge. This was most certainly the case in the Netherlands where until 1870 – when legislation was passed establishing a State Veterinary Service – discussions surrounding meat inspection throughout the mid-nineteenth century had more or less been monopolised by practitioners of human, rather than animal, medicine. Although after this time the issue of food safety continued to be discussed by veterinarians and physicians alike, the state chose the veterinary profession to provide the necessary answers and scientific advice on issues pertaining to meat inspection. The demand for such expertise required that the veterinary curriculum be expanded to prepare aspiring veterinarians for their new role as the caretakers of public health. Hence, in 1881 'practical meat inspection' became a subject in its own right at the Dutch State Veterinary School. Peter Koolmees has in fact argued that official veterinary involvement in meat inspection played a critical role in the social emancipation of the veterinary profession. By entrusting veterinarians with the responsibility for food safety, the profession was further legitimised and its future role as the defender of public health secured (Koolmees 1997: 105–9). In 1919, the veterinary responsibility for public health became firmly embedded in Dutch legislation with the enactment of the Meat Inspection Act (Offringa 1983: 429).

The increasing involvement of the veterinary profession in matters of public health – which culminated in legislation such as the above – bears witness to the increasing formalisation and gradual acceptance of the veterinary regime within western Europe. The role of the veterinarian in protecting and preserving both animal and human health had been firmly established by the turn of the century. Better educated in their art and now equipped with the scientific tools necessary to wage war against animal disease, the profession was finally legitimised by the state and accepted by farmers. The social and political recognition of the veterinary profession had, as this chapter has shown, not been a particularly straightforward business. Most certainly in Britain and the Netherlands, the two emergent industrial nations that have here been discussed, the institutionalisation of the veterinary regime had been fraught with great difficulties that only really began to be properly resolved after the great calamity of the cattle plague. The situation of both these countries perfectly illustrates how industrialisation was accompanied by critical changes in the nature of social relations and an increasing exploitation of animal resources that had in turn led to a situation which necessitated the betterment and intensification of the existing veterinary regime. The veterinary profession had eventually responded to that situation and established itself as a permanent and indispensable fixture within industrial society. In the following chapter, the discussion moves into the twentieth century and considers the far-reaching consequences of the continuing intensification of animal use and the subsequent necessity for the further intensification of the veterinary regime.

5

THE INTENSIFICATION OF LIVESTOCK PRODUCTION AND THE VETERINARY REGIME DURING THE TWENTIETH CENTURY

Down on the farm

The notion of the 'farm' as an idyllic and tranquil place is deeply ingrained in our collective imagination. When we consider the agricultural enterprise, we tend to visualise ruddy-faced 'old Macdonald' herding his cattle through luscious green pastures, hens flapping around the barnyard, curly-tailed pigs wallowing in mud and thatch-roofed cottages. Advertisers and food manufacturers take full advantage of this bucolic imagery when they ply us with 'farm fresh' animal produce and visions of happy, all-dancing and all-singing cows. Urban dwellers flock to the countryside in droves, in search of a rustic escape from the strains and pressures of city life. But what do they find when they arrive? Not always quite what they expect. The picturesque rural landscape has frequently been marred by the presence of obtrusive, cheaply constructed and unattractive industrial-style farm buildings; the good old country smells have been replaced by the unpleasant stench of slurry tanks; and all too often there are few animals to be seen. Bar-coded cattle and sheep may well browse the fields, but the clucking chickens have been cooped up in battery cages and the pigs have all lost their tails to the scalpel. As for 'old Macdonald', the stereotypical country bumpkin farmer has been largely supplanted by the lackeys of big agribusiness (cf. Johnson 1991; Singer 1990).

The conventional image of the agricultural enterprise belies the realities of modern livestock production. It offers a vision of a not too distant past where farming practice had, in essence, changed very little since antiquity. Traditionally, farming had always been a small-scale, and generally family-based, enterprise. Farmers could only keep as many animals as their land could sustain and would generally keep a variety of different species, rather than specialise. Ruminants, such as cattle, sheep and goats, grazed the land; pigs and poultry scavenged and lived off human food scraps. Large-scale livestock production was virtually impossible, because farmers were bound by the size and fertility of the tract of land they owned or rented. Livestock holders had no choice but to use this land to produce animal fodder, which severely restricted the numbers and kinds of animals that they could keep (Schenk 1988: 31). There was also nothing necessarily idyllic or animal friendly about traditional extensive livestock farming practice. Certainly pigs and poultry were allowed to roam free-range, but this was largely due to the fact that animals that foraged for some of their own food were cheaper and easier to maintain (Webster 1994: 134–5).

The nature of agricultural enterprise in the past, much as it is today, was delineated by practical considerations and limitations. Farming methods – e.g. livestock housing systems – were adopted because of the returns that they promised, the manual labour they entailed and the expenses that they were likely to incur. Pragmatic considerations also determined the treatment that livestock received: animals were essentially the farmer's chief asset and their future value would substantially decrease if their welfare was neglected. Farmers then, as now, were therefore impelled to provide their animals with, at the very least, the most basic conditions under which they could yield the produce that would return a profit. Animals that have outlived their usefulness, such as cows too old to breed or milk, have consequently always been most vulnerable to neglect and abuse, whereas young and productive ones have tended to receive the most care (Johnson 1991: 10–11).

The transition from extensive to intensive farming practice

From the late eighteenth century onwards, livestock production began to change significantly. The massive growth in human population and animal food demands during the late eighteenth and nineteenth centuries led to the increasing intensification of animal use throughout Europe. Agrarian developments, such as land enclosure in Britain and the introduction of fodder crops in the

Netherlands, provided the initial impetus for changes in animal husbandry. Ruminants kept in enclosures, rather than on common land, no longer had to be so hardy to survive and experimental breeding began in order to produce larger and better quality animals. Likewise, growing crops, such as turnips, for fodder allowed for indoor feeding. It therefore became economically viable for farmers to keep more non-breeding animals alive during the harsh winter months. In this way, meat was no longer necessarily a seasonal luxury and could be consumed all year round, particularly by the more affluent (Johnson 1991: 12, 56). The demand for food of animal origin continued to increase with the rapid expansion of the human population and the gradual improvement of the standard of living, while the number of people actually involved in agriculture and animal husbandry steadily declined as people migrated to urban areas. As the processes of industrialisation and urbanisation got under way, commerce and manufacturing rapidly overtook agriculture as the primary source of wealth.

Farmers, however, often found themselves unable to cope with the ever-increasing food demands of the rapidly expanding populations of western Europe. Their solution – as illustrated in the previous chapter – was to import stock from the distant and more thinly populated lands of eastern Europe where food-producing animals were cheap and abundant; or alternatively, to import meat from Australia and New Zealand. The infrastructural and technological developments of the industrial age made animal transportation a viable option and the movement of both live animals and animal produce across increasingly greater distances became commonplace. One of the main consequences of these new animal markets was that European nations began to experience a far greater degree of economic interdependence than ever before. For example, during the mid-nineteenth century, Britain – the fastest growing industrial power – increasingly came to depend on the import of beef, pork and lamb from the Netherlands and Denmark. Dutch livestock producers, in turn, attempted to intensify and modify their production and breeding methods in order to produce meat that would most greatly appeal to the demands and appetites of their neighbours (Davids 1989: 84–5). However, although there were clear moves to intensify livestock production, farmers were still very much constrained in the numbers and types of animals they could keep by the acreage and yield of their own land. Extensive farming methods thus continued to provide the agricultural norm up until the mid-twentieth century.

The twentieth century has in fact borne witness to the most radical and rapid transformation of livestock production methods in agricultural history. During the post-war period, the traditional face of European agriculture changed almost irrevocably as alternative systems of animal management were developed allowing large numbers of animals to be kept and maintained with the minimum of labour (costs). Population dynamics have in part been responsible for the rapid intensification of livestock production. The ever-growing and increasingly more affluent urban populations have demanded increasingly more animal produce at affordable prices. Meat, in particular, has become a dietary staple. Since the Second World War, the consumption of animal flesh, dairy produce and eggs has increased in keeping with intensive growth. While the urban populace has continued to expand, the numbers of people involved in agricultural production have steadily declined leaving fewer people to work the land and maintain livestock. This demographic change and increased consumer demand is, of course, a continuation of the nineteenth-century situation. However, unlike their predecessors who were necessarily restricted to employing extensive farming methods, modern livestock producers have been liberated from the shackles of their land by a new industrial development; namely, the evolution of the animal feed industry.

The modern animal feed industry presented farmers with the possibility of keeping far more livestock than their own land could sustain for it provided them with an external source of fodder, freeing precious land for other purposes. Moreover, it gave farmers the ideal opportunity to greatly increase production to meet growing consumer demands for animal produce. The main impetus for the development of this new industry was the crisis faced by European agriculture during the late nineteenth century. Between 1878 and 1895, grain exports from the Ukraine and North America led to a huge drop in grain prices. Prices continued to remain low, eventually leading to the use of cheap grain as animal feed (Bieleman 1992: 214–17). Throughout the twentieth century, the animal feed industry has continued to play a significant role in the development of intensive livestock farming methods, particularly with regard to the design of livestock housing and the introduction of automated feeding systems. The increasing mechanisation of agriculture, allowing animal feed and manure to be moved in vast quantities, has also been a major factor in the intensification of livestock farming. Livestock production has become an increasingly profitable business since the Second World War, particularly given the governmental subsidies and banking loans that farmers have received in order to increase productivity. Such external funding has greatly benefited farmers and has allowed them to make the move from extensive to intensive livestock production, providing them with the capital necessary to make investments in new buildings, livestock housing systems and automated agricultural equipment. The financiers of modern agribusiness have, as a consequence, wielded a considerable amount of power and influence on the nature and future of agricultural development (Schenk 1988: 34–5).

The labour costs involved in producing livestock have also increased in relation to the costs of animal feed, fuel, housing and equipment; this is mainly due to the increase in consumer incomes and spending power (Webster 1994: 135). However, largely by replacing a human workforce with mechanised and automated systems, both labour and production costs have been significantly reduced. Livestock are fed mechanically and, in many housing systems, animal waste is conveyed away automatically, saving farm workers both time and energy and farm owners wage bills. The decision to specialise in the intensive production of one species, often for very specific purposes such as egg, milk, or meat production, has greatly simplified the business of livestock production and has reduced labour costs (Schenk 1988: 34–5). Webster argues that by choosing to intensify livestock production and providing new housing systems, farmers have been driven to stock animals as densely as possible, in order to maximise their output relative to the cost of the buildings and equipment they have acquired and to reduce feed costs by minimising the animals' expenditure of energy in activity and keeping warm (Webster 1994: 135). The upshot of such choices are the 'factory farms' that are characteristic of modern agricultural production.

In addition to the aforementioned economic and demographic factors, two scientific and technological developments of the twentieth century have permitted food-producing animals to be housed indoors in such great densities. First, the harnessing of electrical power and the eventual post-war connection of farms to national electricity grids enabled livestock producers to use artificial light, employ cooling and heating systems to assist and stimulate animal production (Johnson 1991: 27). Electricity also provided the means by which the automation of feeding systems, etc., could be realised. Secondly, veterinary and pharmaceutical advances made it possible and safer to stock animals at higher densities. Although – as will be discussed shortly – modern farming systems still pose potentially serious health risks for both animals and humans, infectious animal disease can to a large extent be controlled by routine vaccination and the widespread use of antibiotics, particularly in feed. In recent years, immunological and biotechnological research has played an increasingly important role in the development of vaccines, reproduction technology and animal nutrition. Such scientific advancement has further assisted livestock producers in the efficient production of healthy stock that can be converted into animal protein in sufficient quantities and at an acceptable price and quality for the consumer.

The transition from extensive to intensive farming practices has been exceptionally rapid. Since the 1950s, livestock production in some parts of Europe has been transformed almost beyond recognition. Some of the technology and systems employed in modern livestock production have, however, been in existence for much longer. As Thomas reveals, during the sixteenth century, pigs were kept in 'sweat-boxes' so small that they could not turn around, being forced to lie on their abdomens. Poultry were similarly fattened in dark confinement and lambs specially reared for the yuletide feasts of the nobility in small dark cabins (Thomas 1983: 94). During the nineteenth century, veal producers in the Netherlands fattened calves on sweet milk in pens so small that the animals could barely move. They were kept for a period of twelve to thirteen weeks, reaching an average weight of 30 to 40 kilos at slaughter (Davids 1989: 73–4).[1] Similarly, the wire mesh technology used in battery production has existed for over 100 years and patents on battery cages have been taken out since the 1920s (Johnson 1991: 27). The potential for and desirability of intensive farming has, therefore, perhaps always been there. It is simply the suitable technological and economic conditions for the widespread housing of livestock in small spaces and high densities – and the veterinary care for them – that have been lacking in the past.

During the 1930s, the most decisive moves towards the intensification of livestock farming occurred in the United States with the introduction of the battery system of poultry production. During the post-war period, European farmers followed suit and instigated the transition from extensive to intensive livestock production. In the Netherlands, for example, the intensification of farming had a fairly late start, beginning properly only in the 1960s. Intensive systems of livestock production presented Dutch farmers with a particularly attractive proposition at a time in which the demand for and price of land for the construction of housing, roads and industrial developments was steadily rising. The new livestock housing systems entailed an enormous saving for farmers in terms of the space and capital necessary to increase productivity (de Waal 1987: 59). Despite a slow start, since that time the Netherlands has become perhaps the most intensively farmed country in Europe and has moved to the forefront of livestock production technology. To illustrate this, the agricultural census of 1996 revealed that this small country – with a human population of 15 million people – was home to approximately 14.4 million pigs, 4.55 million cattle and 91 million chickens, not to mention hundreds of thousands of sheep, goats and other farm animals and several million pets (Centraal Bureau voor Statistiek 1996).

The move towards intensive farming has in fact had a colossal effect on the whole enterprise of farming. As Singer (1990) suggests, agriculture has today been transformed into agribusiness. For example, in 1950 there were 1.8 million pigs in the Netherlands, twenty-five years later this figure had increased four-fold. Yet, in spite of this huge increase in animals, there were far fewer farming operatives engaged in pig farming and breeding; in 1960, there were 150,000 Dutch farms specialising in pig production, as compared with 50,000 during the 1970s (Davids 1989: 73–4). In the United States, agribusiness is even more concentrated with, for example, fifty large corporations controlling virtually all poultry production. Competitors have been forced to adopt the same methods as the big producers, or else go out of business (Singer 1990: 96). Such competition has in fact been one of the most important driving forces in the spread of intensive methods of livestock farming. In turn, the spread of these new farming methods and competition between livestock producers have improved the availability and reduced the cost of animal produce; a development to which both consumers and retailers have responded favourably, leading to a great rise in the sale and consumption of the products derived from the new livestock industry (Webster 1994: 135). Clearly the intensification of livestock production has had significant consequences for the whole nature of the agricultural enterprise and the people and animals involved in it. This chapter will consider the ramifications of intensive farming still further with regard to animal welfare, the environment and public health. The second half will be devoted to the discussion of large-animal medicine during the twentieth century and how it has responded to the very new challenges to animal well-being and public health that the increasing exploitation of animal resources through new farming methods have presented.

Animal welfare: poultry, pigs and cattle

As the above discussion suggests, the intensification of livestock production has been accompanied by significant changes in both the numbers and kinds of animals kept and the conditions under which they live. Take, for example, the humble chicken. Once upon a time, domestic fowl either scavenged freely around the farmyard, or were kept in open runs or small huts. Such birds were highly vulnerable to predators, exposure to disease and climatic conditions. Moreover, they consumed large quantities of food, while laying far fewer eggs than they were physically capable of producing. Commercially, keeping poultry in this fashion was not particularly profitable since not all eggs laid would necessarily be found or be fresh when collected (Sainsbury 1986: 156). During the 1920s, the first experimental systems of intensive poultry keeping were developed, eventually leading to the commercial production of battery cages in 1930 (Ryder 1989: 262). The modern battery housing system that derives from these experiments has today become the epitome of efficient intensive livestock production systems and has been widely adopted throughout the industrial world.

Battery chickens are confined indoors, crammed into small and barren wire cages and stacked in tiers along the walls of long, windowless buildings. Each cage – with the approximate dimensions of 40cm x 50cm x 40cm – is home to four or five chickens; birds housed individually tend to lay less prolifically and take up too much space. The floors of the cages slope, in order that the eggs the birds lay will roll forward onto a rack or conveyor belt. Food is supplied mechanically and the birds' droppings will fall into a pit below the cages, or will be spirited away by another conveyor belt. The chickens are routinely vaccinated against infectious disease via their drinking water or through the use of aerosols. Artificial lighting and temperature controls ensure that the birds will lay eggs all year round (Johnson 1991: 27). The chickens – hatched in incubators especially for this purpose – are placed in these battery cages at about twenty weeks of age and will remain there for around fourteen months, after which their productivity is reduced and they will be replaced by new birds. Each bird will lay, on average, 5 eggs a week, producing approximately 300 eggs during this fourteen-month period (de Waal 1987: 60–1). This is in sharp contrast to the layer hens of the 1930s that produced an average of 121 eggs per annum (Mason and Singer 1980: 41). Today, in Britain, the Netherlands and the United States, ninety per cent of egg-laying flocks are kept in battery cages (Johnson 1991; de Waal 1987). The battery system has been so universally embraced by farmers because it has provided them with the possibility of mechanising their operations, thereby reducing labour costs and profitably keeping large numbers of birds in a restricted space.

The demand for poultry meat has greatly increased since the Second World War. As the popularity of red meat has declined and the costs of poultry production have fallen, chicken has enjoyed increasing popularity in the western diet. Billions of chickens are slaughtered each year on the abattoir conveyor belt in order to meet the consumer clamour for white meat; and it is the modern farming industry that makes it possible for them to afford it. The lot of broiler chickens (i.e. birds destined for the table) is not too different from their egg-laying relatives, though instead of being housed in cages, they are usually crammed – as day-old chicks – in their thousands onto the floor of a huge shed strewn with litter. Their environment is completely controlled in order to make them grow faster and fatter for the dinner plate with as little feed as possible. As they rapidly grow, the hens' living space becomes increasingly more overcrowded. When the birds are ripe for slaughter, at about six to seven weeks old, the sheds are cleared and disinfected ready for the next delivery of chicks from the hatchery. In contrast, the natural life-span of a chicken is approximately seven *years* (Singer 1990: 98–9). Broiler chickens have been genetically selected and bred to grow rapidly, particularly the succulent white breast muscle that is so favoured by consumers (Webster 1994: 155–6).[2] Poultry breeders have been extraordinarily successful in producing birds that grow at a phenomenal rate and yield cheap white meat. During the mid-1960s, it took a broiler chicken at least fourteen weeks to reach the slaughter weight that a bird today will grow to within seven (Johnson 1991: 30). Turkeys are kept and reared in a similar fashion.

Rearing and keeping poultry in such a fashion has not been without its problems. The first farmers who attempted to crowd large flocks into confined, and often inadequately ventilated, spaces soon discovered that infectious diseases spread rapidly amongst flocks resulting in high mortality amongst birds and heavy financial losses. Furthermore, they found that, in these crowded conditions, some birds would peck others to death and even consume their remains (Mason and Singer 1980: 1–2). Chickens are, by nature, highly social creatures that develop and live within a hierarchical social order, commonly referred to as a 'pecking order'. When chickens are crowded together in such high densities, they are unable to establish a social order amongst themselves and resort to feather-pecking and cannibalism. Such 'vices', as they are referred to by poultry producers, ultimately cost farmers money. But instead of reducing overcrowding – thus reducing the stress suffered by the birds – poultry farmers have generally opted to tackle the problem of the damage caused by aggressive behaviour at the very source: the beak.

'Debeaking' fowl to prevent birds from picking at each other's feathers is a technique that was developed during the 1940s. Originally, this procedure was performed using a blowtorch; today, a guillotine-style device using hot blades has been developed for this purpose (Singer 1990: 99–101). Debeaking is a procedure that is generally performed soon after the chicks are hatched; it removes a sensitive part of the bird's beak and can impair its ability to select and pick at food (Sainsbury 1986: 82–3). Trimming the birds' beaks, however, does not deal with the underlying cause of this abnormal behaviour, namely overcrowding and boredom. Reduction in overcrowding would necessarily mean a reduction in the profit margins for poultry producers, and is therefore not expedient. A further attempt to reduce the aggression of birds, particularly as they reach slaughter weight and their living space is extremely cramped, is to keep them in dimly lit surroundings. Exposure to light, or a lack thereof, is an important factor in the growth and development of broiler chickens. The addition of the vitamins A and D, minerals and antibiotics to the birds' feed means that sunlight and exercise are no longer essential to ensure growth and bone development in poultry (Mason and Singer 1980: 1).

Further to this, the deliberate breeding and genetic selection of broiler chickens for rapid growth and grossly enlarged breast muscle has had serious consequences for the health and welfare of poultry. Birds can suffer from a variety of pathological conditions of bones, joints, tendons and skin, generally referred to under the general epithet of 'leg weakness'. The leg movement of fowl can be impaired as birds grow too heavy for their limbs, or become too physically distorted, thereby placing unnatural stresses on their joints. The chief repercussion of this is that the birds will spend a considerable portion of their already short lives in chronic pain (Webster 1994: 156). Likewise, battery hens may suffer a degree of physical discomfort and pain in the conditions under which they live. Barren wire cages can damage the birds' feet and feathers, and they do not have any exercise. Moreover, inadequate nutrition may lead to osteoporosis, ultimately resulting in bone weakness and fractures. The battery system greatly restricts the birds' natural behaviour: they cannot adequately preen their feathers or stretch their limbs, nor can they turn around properly. Aggression and feather-pecking is therefore a problem amongst battery layer chickens. Battery-caged fowl cannot clean themselves naturally, for they have no litter or dust to bathe in. The way in which cages are stacked means that it is difficult for all birds to be adequately inspected for injury or health problems. Moreover, the reliance on automated systems to maintain virtually all aspects of the feeding and maintenance of the birds has serious welfare implications if such systems fail (Sainsbury 1986: 160).

The rise of modern poultry farming has been phenomenal. It has almost completely supplanted the traditional methods of poultry rearing, leading to a massive increase in the consumption – and decrease in the price – of chicken since the Second World War. In this respect, poultry farming is quite unique. Although 'factory farming' systems have been adopted for the production of other livestock species, they continue to coexist with other traditional or less intensive methods of animal husbandry (Johnson 1991: 34). Next to chickens, pigs are the species that are most widely subjected to intensive farming methods. Traditionally, pigs were housed in sties, with access to an outside yard where they could exercise, feed, drink and defecate. Modern piggeries are a far cry from tradition, although there is a great deal of variation in the degree of confinement and environment in which modern commercially farmed pigs will live. Some pig farms, however, bear close resemblance to the poultry production units described above. These are large and highly automated farms that have been specially designed to rear pigs in total confinement. Pigs are thus born, weaned and fattened for slaughter without ever seeing the direct light of day. The environment with which the pig is provided is designed entirely to maximise profit and minimise labour costs. The pig's naturally prolific reproductive and growth cycles are exploited to their very limits (Mason and Singer 1980: 8).

Pregnant sows will often spend the entire sixteen-week gestation period confined to an individual – concrete or slatted-floored – narrow stall in which they can sit and stand, but not turn around. Such stalls, or alternatively the tethering of pigs, allow farmers to use floor space more efficiently and keep larger numbers of pigs under one roof. Before they give birth, sows are moved to special farrowing crates where they are kept in a position from which their piglets can easily be suckled. These crates are designed not only to reduce the risk of the sow lying on her progeny and crushing them, but also to allow the stockman safe access to them. Piglets remain with their mothers for about three weeks, after which they are removed to artificially heated group pens to be fattened for slaughter. To prevent further lactation, the sow is denied food and water for twenty-four hours, returned to the breeding area where she is served by a boar, beginning the whole cycle anew. Apart from those kept for breeding purposes, the young pigs will be kept for between four and six months until they reach the slaughter weight desirable for either pork or bacon production. Young pigs are often stocked at high densities in dimly lit conditions in order that they gain weight rapidly with as little exercise as possible. Sometimes sweat boxes are used to attain this same goal (Johnson 1991: 35). Antibiotics are commonly employed in the animals' feed, not only to prevent disease but also to promote growth. The growing pigs often live in a barren environment, on concrete or slatted floors that are easy to maintain. Such flooring, however, can result in joint disorders, lameness and injury for the animals. The absence of straw, while more convenient for maintenance and sanitation, prevents pigs from being able to perform their natural rooting behaviour. Pigs kept in total confinement, without stimulation, have a tendency to suffer great stress and boredom. Supporters of intensive pig farming have, however, claimed that these living conditions lead to increased productivity, improved disease control, better sanitation and greater general efficiency in swine management and production (Tannenbaum 1989: 253–4). Such commercial systems of pig production have indeed reduced the price of pig meat and consumers have responded favourably.

Like broiler chickens, the overcrowded conditions in which pigs are kept can lead to aggression and injury. To prevent cannibalism and tail-biting injuries, piglets kept in such total confinement have their needle-like teeth clipped and tails docked. It is also common practice in pig farming for virtually all male pigs, apart from those used for breeding, to be castrated between the approximate age of seven and fourteen days. The rationale behind this is that castration prevents the animal's flesh from being tainted by an unpleasant taste and boar odour, which is offensive to many consumers and would render the pig's flesh unsaleable. The export of meat from uncastrated pigs is also not permitted under European Union (EU) regulations and can only be used in the production of meat products under very specific conditions (de Waal 1987: 82). Castrated animals are perceived to be less aggressive and easier to handle. Moreover, they tend to grow faster and yield more (less fatty) meat. Although this practice is more or less ubiquitous to swine management, it is widely criticised as an unnecessary mutilation that incurs unnecessarily high costs for pig production (Tannenbaum 1989: 253). Pig castration is considered by many to be both cruel and unnecessary for two main reasons: first, the way in which it is sometimes performed – as described below – is believed to cause pain and stress for the animals (Broom and Johnson 1993: 91) and second, it has been argued that it is pointless, most particularly in view of intensive factory farming production, because few pigs ever reach maturity and most are sent to the slaughterhouses at too young an age for the adult hormones which might taint the flesh to be activated (Johnson 1991: 131). In view of this, in 1987 the European Parliament adopted a policy towards animal welfare and intensive farming methods which recommended that this practice, amongst others, be stopped (Singer 1990: 143–4). The Dutch government, in particular, has been a chief advocate in the need to change the EU's policy on the castration of piglets. They argue that meat contaminated with boar taint could instead be detected by abattoir controls and meat inspection (Ministerie van Landbouw, Natuurbeheer en Visserij 1992: 13–14). The only benefit that this practice has to offer is that it renders pigs more profitable, tractable and easier for farmers to manage.

Traditional piglet castration – certainly as I have seen it practised in the Netherlands – is performed entirely without anaesthetic. The piglets are held up in the air by their hind legs and the scrotum is sliced open to expose the testicles, which are then pulled out and swiftly removed using a scalpel. Still held upside down, a diluted iodine solution is splashed on their behinds to sterilise the wound. From their behavioural responses and vocalisation, it is apparent that castration causes the piglets pain and distress. Although piglets have a tendency to squeal loudly when handled, it has been established that the frequency of their screams is in fact far higher during castration. Moreover, it has been demonstrated that the discomfort caused can continue for several days after the actual castration has occurred (Broom and Johnson 1993: 91). Experiments with and without the use of local anaesthetic have indicated that castrating piglets without causes them greater stress (White *et al.* 1995).

Further to this, piglet castration brings with it the chance of infection, e.g. abscesses, tetanus and the spread of infectious diseases such as classical swine fever, from the implements used (de Waal 1987: 82). Although opposed by the European Parliament, this procedure is perfectly legal and does not even have to be performed by a trained vet. In the Netherlands, this practice is sometimes performed by specialist para-veterinarians known as castrators, but also by unqualified farmers. It is an unrestricted practice that can be performed regardless of the age and size of the pig, although it is habitually done at the age of seven to fourteen days. Anaesthetic is too costly, requires the skills of a trained vet and there is always the risk that the animal might die as a result.

The plight of poultry and pigs has to some extent been shared by cattle, although the fact that cattle still roam green pastures somewhat obscures the extent to which mechanisation and intensification have affected these ruminants. Yet it was the predicament of veal calves that led to the initial outcry and concern for the welfare of food-producing animals back in the 1960s. The defenceless brown-eyed calf confined to a small dark crate, as described by Harrison in the book *Animal Machines* (1964), came to symbolise the cruelty of modern livestock production in the public eye. In order to produce the tender, pale flesh that the gourmet consumer desires, calves are taken from their mothers just a few days after they are born and are put into small wooden crates. For fourteen to sixteen weeks, they are fed – twice a day – on a mixture of dried skimmed milk, dried whey, starch, fats, sugar, vitamins, minerals and antibiotics (Mason and Singer 1980: 13). This diet has been specially formulated to be high in fat and deficient in iron. The animal is almost completely immobilised, the restriction of movement and diet leads to anaemia and consequently the production of white flesh. The calves miss their mothers and cannot be suckled, they cannot turn properly in order to groom themselves, nor are they permitted to ruminate since roughage contains iron and that would darken the flesh. They are kept in darkness, except during feeding times, and are deprived of visual stimulation and contact with other calves (Singer 1990: 132–5). Pneumonia and diarrhoea are also common to calves kept in these conditions (de Waal 1987: 70). The lot of the veal calf is a far from happy one and in view of this, this method of rearing calves has been prohibited in the United Kingdom. The veal crate, however, is still in common use throughout the rest of Europe and the United States; although it must be noted that in recent years the practice of rearing calves in groups rather than isolation seems to be becoming increasingly prevalent. Much of the veal produced in Europe comes from calves originally exported from Britain. These calves are reared in neighbouring lands, such as the Netherlands, who in turn export the veal to countries like Italy and France where white flesh is in the most demand.

The increasing consumer demand for milk and dairy produce has largely been responsible for the rise of the veal industry. To ensure that dairy cows produce milk, they must produce a calf each year. The calf is then removed from the mother, otherwise it would consume the milk from which the farmer will make his profit. These calves will either be destined for veal production, or they will be fed on milk substitutes and reared to be dairy calves, or fattened as beef cattle (Singer 1990: 136). Although the majority of European cattle still graze outdoors – only being brought into the byre for winter shelter and to avoid damage to grass during rainy periods – cattle are increasingly being confined indoors as farmers employ their land to produce silage for feed: this is known as 'zero-grazing'. The conditions under which such cattle live vary considerably according to the housing system adopted by the farmer: they may be tethered, or live in cubicle-style housing. Dairy cattle can sometimes move freely around their stalling, but this also can be too crowded. The local availability of straw influences the living conditions of cattle. Using straw for bedding is more labour intensive, therefore cattle are nowadays kept on flooring of bare concrete or wooden slats (Johnson 1991: 38). Slatted floors are less comfortable for cattle to lie on and can contribute to foot injuries and lameness.

The confinement of cattle to indoor stalls has brought with it a need for a surgical intervention akin to the debeaking of chickens and docking of pigs' tails. The high densities in which cattle are housed has led to the necessity of the routine removal of the animals' horns. Injuries occur as cattle jab each other while sorting out their social hierarchies. Dairy cattle are therefore habitually 'dehorned' to prevent the goring of other cattle and their human handlers. Injury would involve more expense and possible loss of productivity for the farmers. Dehorning is usually performed on young calves whose horns have not yet developed. It involves burning out the root of the horn, under mild anaesthesia, so that blood vessels and nerve endings are sealed off and horn growth is prevented. Hair and skin will eventually grow over the burned area and will, after a few days, cause the animal no further discomfort. There is consensus amongst veterinarians that this is the kindest way of removing horns. Sawing them off later is perceived to be more painful and traumatic for the animal, although burning them out inflicts a degree of pain and stress. Dehorning adult cattle, however, is not only believed to be painful, but it can impede milk productivity (Tannenbaum 1989: 257).

The quest for increasingly higher milk yields has led to significant changes in the lives of dairy cattle. Like poultry and pigs, the cow's environment and diet are controlled with the sole purpose of maximising milk yield in mind. In order to increase output, cattle are given high-energy supplementary feeds containing, for instance, silage, soya-beans, fishmeal or brewing by-products (Singer 1990: 137). Also, the (inadequately sterilised) rendered-down by-products of slaughter such as sheep's brains have been included in these feeds. The wisdom thereof has been dramatically challenged by the emergence of bovine spongiform encephalopathy, a horrifying new disease of cattle, in Britain during the late 1980s. Such diets are not entirely appropriate to the cow's unique digestive system and can result in the development of a condition known as rumen acidosis, leading to discomfort and even lameness. The inclusion of silage in the cow's diet can increase the risk of mastitis, i.e. the inflammation of the udder (Johnson 1991: 40). With such problems in mind, trials have been conducted in recent years using a recombinant bovine growth hormone, known as bovine somatotropin (BST), in order to further increase milk yields. This synthetic hormone increases 'the capacity of the mammary gland to synthesise milk without adjusting the anatomical or physical ability of the cow to process nutrients' (Webster 1994: 172). Neither the effects on the health of cattle nor the negative effects of residues of this hormone on humans have yet been quantified. Its use has not yet been permitted within the European Union, though it is currently being employed in the United States. In short, all attempts today are directed to working dairy cattle to the very limits of their productivity and beyond.

Cattle intended for beef production in Europe share similar living conditions to those of dairy cattle, being kept in outdoor pastures or indoor stalling. In the USA, however, they are often housed in vast 'feedlots' where stocking densities are high and the environment barren (Singer 1990: 140). The chief welfare concern with regard to beef cattle is that of breeding practices. The most important by-product of the beef cow is, of course, her calf. Attempts to increase the size of calves and impose twin births have created serious problems for the beef cow. Obstetric difficulties are today part and parcel of the business of beef production. Calves – especially double-muscled breeds such as the Belgian Blue – can be deliberately bred too large to be born naturally and must, therefore, be delivered by caesarean section. Cows are subjected to repeated caesareans during their lifetimes which, although conducted under local anaesthetic, can lead to residual pain. The issue is not whether or not the operation should be performed at all – from a veterinary perspective it is essential to try to save two lives – but whether it is ethically acceptable that calves must almost inevitably be born in this way, and the health of their mothers be endangered as a consequence, as a result of breeding practices which produce unnaturally heavy and large calves designed specifically for meat production (Rutgers 1993: 159–69). The embryo transfers, which often result in such births, can in themselves create potential health problems for the beef cow (Webster 1994: 184–5).

The housing and treatment of livestock has been a major concern of animal rights and animal welfare organisations in recent years. There are grave concerns that intensive livestock production violates the most basic rights of agricultural animals; namely that animals must have sufficient freedom of movement to be able to stand up, lie down, groom themselves normally, to turn around and stretch their limbs properly. In other words, that the most basic natural behaviour of animals should be respected. As the above discussion has illustrated, animals kept in great concentrations in dull and 'unnatural' surroundings have a tendency to display aberrant behaviour. This has led to 'mutilations', such as debeaking, tail-docking and dehorning, becoming common practice, for they help to prevent unnecessary injury to both the animals and the farmer's pocket. These mutilations are often perceived as cruel and are condemned because they ignore the underlying cause of the animals' aggression towards one another.

The proponents of animal rights believe that – if animals should be kept for food at all – they should be afforded living conditions roughly similar to the animal's natural habitat. However, as Sainsbury (1986) points out, the well-meaning can be rather myopic in their determination to create alternative, 'natural' livestock production systems. Although free-range animals – in contrast to their 'factory-farmed' cousins – can move around with ease in a 'natural' setting, their health – and thus welfare – is often at stake given their exposure to stress and harm from bad weather, be it cold, wet or excessively warm; not to mention their lack of protection from predators (e.g. dogs, foxes, etc.) and disease which can result in serious losses and a fall in productivity. In contrast, indoor livestock production units should – at least in theory – be able to provide a controlled environment where disease can be monitored and both vermin and predators excluded. Furthermore, the treatment that animals receive from the stockmen who attend to them has a bearing on the welfare and productivity of livestock. If the animals are fearful of the people with whom they come into contact, their level of stress increases. It has been found that the attitudes and behaviour of stockmen towards farm animals have a significant impact on their welfare and productivity (Hemsworth *et al*. 1993).

Thus, both free range and intensive farming have their limitations with respect to animal welfare, disease control and productivity. Ultimately, our society's demand for a constant supply of affordable animal produce of a standard quality is responsible for the rise of the intensive systems of livestock production that are today vilified for their cruelty and inhumanity. Consumers seem to be becoming increasingly aware of and interested in the circumstances of food production, to some extent leading to a growing concern for animal welfare and an increasing demand for animal produce that has been produced in a more 'animal-friendly' fashion, although it should be added that criticism of farming methods and actual consumer behaviour do not necessarily go hand in hand. Alternative systems of livestock housing are currently being developed that will still afford farmers a high level of productivity and profit, while providing the animals with a more stimulating and humane environment. It remains to be seen what the future holds.

The environmental impact of intensive livestock production

The intensification of livestock production has had not only a significant effect on animal welfare, but also a considerable impact on the environment. In this regard, the disposal of the enormous quantities of animal waste produced by animals confined in intensive livestock production units has created the greatest environmental problems (El-Ahraf and Willis 1996: 1–28). The reduction of manpower levels and the need for efficient animal management have meant that 'factory' farmers have often abandoned the use of straw as bedding in livestock houses; the animals instead stand on slatted or solid concrete floors. The faeces and urine which these animals produce must therefore be disposed of differently. When straw bedding is used, manure is collected in dung heaps, exposed to air it gradually ferments, bacteria are thus to some extent destroyed and the excreta eventually becomes fertiliser to be spread on the land. Slurry, on the other hand, must be stored in tanks, where it may decompose and sometimes produce a variety of noxious smelling gases. This method does not kill pathogens quite as effectively as the traditional method (Johnson 1991: 144–5). While straw bedding most closely resembles the natural surface on which most animals lie – and is thus promoted as the ideal floor surface on which animals should be kept – it can provide the conditions under which disease organisms can flourish. If poorly maintained, such bedding when excessively dirty and wet not only causes distress to the animals, but can also lead to environmental mastitis in dairy cattle, 'farrowing fever' in pregnant sows and an increased exposure of poultry to the dangerous *E. coli* bacteria (Sainsbury 1986: 70).

Slurry can be returned to the land as fertiliser, but its storage and application can be particularly problematic. It cannot be spread when the ground is too wet and must, therefore, be stored in huge tanks, sometimes for several months. The failure of these storage tanks would have a significant impact on the local environment, most particularly if pathogens, such as salmonella, *E. coli* and leptospira, which are dangerous to both human and animal health, were still present in the slurry. To reduce the risk of infection, farmers have been warned against spreading slurry on grazing land. If they must do so, they are advised to allow the slurry to adequately ferment and to leave the land on which it has been spread unpastured for at least six weeks afterwards (Johnson 1991: 147–8). The main problem with modern farms is that they do not always have enough land to absorb the waste that the animals produce. The waste must, therefore, often be transported elsewhere at considerable expense to the livestock holder. As Johnson (1991) suggests, waste disposal can be the main factor which determines how many animals can viably be kept in a livestock production unit, rather than animal welfare. To illustrate this problem, he describes the crisis faced in the Netherlands during the late 1980s. The great concentration of factory farms had put so much pressure on land that by January 1987 the Dutch authorities placed a ban on the further expansion of livestock numbers. With farms producing around 100 million tonnes of effluent per annum, twice the amount of liquid waste accumulated than could safely be spread on the country's 2 million hectares of farmland. As a consequence, the transport of slurry to areas away from factory farms was encouraged and subsidised by the Dutch government and large-scale dumping of slurry was banned due to the potential pollution and health risks it presented. Dutch farmers are now required to pay the full costs of disposal through sewage plants if they are unable to find appropriate land to spread their farm waste on (Johnson 1991: 149).

Like slurry, the production of silage – a grass crop harvested when green and then partially fermented to make animal fodder – can present serious environmental problems. The anaerobic fermentation which accompanies silage production can potentially produce a waste liquid which has been estimated to be 200 times more polluting than domestic sewage, particularly when the grass is wet. Such waste presents great pollution problems if it escapes the silos in which it is held and enters natural waterways. The aquatic life of rivers and streams can be either poisoned or starved of oxygen as a result of the introduction of this effluent (Johnson 1991: 146). The contamination of natural waterways is one of the most serious environmental consequences of modern agricultural practice. Aside from the problems posed by slurry and silage effluent, intensive livestock production contributes towards nitrate pollution (El-Ahraf and Willis 1996: 16–17). In addition to this, the additives used in animal feed and the antibiotics which the animals are routinely given are potential sources of environmental contamination. Although the blame for environmental pollution is often apportioned to industry, rather than agriculture, the intensification of farming methods – most particularly with respect to the waste it produces – presents a significant threat to the environment.

Intensive livestock production: disease risks, control and prevention

In addition to the phenomenal impact on animal welfare and the environment, the intensification of livestock production has created new opportunities for disease organisms to flourish and threaten the health of both animal and human populations. As this book has thus far clearly illustrated, our interactions with other animals have always brought with them the potential risk of infectious disease. However, the increasing exploitation of and dependency on animal resources, that has occurred through the intensification of livestock production, has meant that disease *risks* which did not exist, or were unthinkable, forty to fifty years ago are today commonplace. In short, the increase in stocking densities has led to the increase of opportunities for disease transmission.

The housing and living conditions of intensively farmed animals – most notably pigs and poultry – potentially provide significant exposure to bacteria and viruses, thereby enhancing the risk of disease. Disease risks can be greatly reduced with good stockmanship. On 'factory farms', however, animal management is primarily linked to maintaining or increasing productivity. In the past, stockmen could attend to animals more individually and were familiar with the small herds they tended. Today, stockmen are not only fewer in number, but are also required to manage huge numbers of livestock as efficiently and cost effectively as possible. The reduction of manpower levels in livestock farming combined with the increasing numbers of animals kept on site can lead to inefficiency in disease control and hygiene which, in turn, may result in the outbreak of infectious disease amongst the animal stock and – depending on the nature of the disease in question – possibly even transmission to the humans who come into direct contact with them. This is, of course, not to mention the risk of contaminated animal protein entering into the food chain and putting human consumers at risk of infection (Brander and Ellis 1977; Johnson 1991; Sainsbury 1986).

One of the disease management techniques adopted in intensive livestock production is to accept the pervasiveness of infection. Antibiotic drugs and vaccinations are thus routinely administered in order to keep stock healthy and maintain productivity. When disease outbreaks occur, it may not be viable to cull stock given the size of the animal population housed. Similarly, farm buildings may have been too poorly constructed and cannot be properly disinfected or cleaned, the animal's excreta, as suggested above, creating potential hazards for both animal and public health. Management of disease purely through drug intervention is far from ideal. Moreover, it arouses considerable consumer concern about the quality of the animal produce which ends up on our dinner plates. The use of growth hormones and the possibly harmful effects of veterinary drug residues in food have become an increasing source of consumer anxiety in recent years; as has the suggestion that the persistent administration of antibiotic drugs may ultimately lead to the evolution of pathogens resistant to such substances (Sainsbury 1986: 5–6).

For fifty years, antibiotics have been added to animal feeds in order to improve feeding efficiency and growth rates. Since the

1960s, scientists have looked into the possibilities of resistance risks and by 1970 the European community had made moves to prevent the antibiotics that are used in human medicine being used as animal growth promoters. Today, the issue of resistant risks has again become the topic of political and scientific debate, stimulated in part by the development of a veterinary antibiotic called *avoparcin* which is closely related to an important human medical antibiotic known as *vancomycin.* There is a concern that such veterinary antibiotics may promote the emergence of bacterial strains that have a genetic resistance to antibiotics. Although there is currently little microbiological consensus on this topic, some scientists have gone so far as to suggest that the widespread use of antibiotics in livestock production, particularly those used to treat infections, may well be responsible for resistant strains of salmonella and campylobacter that are being found in increasing numbers of food poisoning cases in humans (Bonner 1997). In recent years, the problem of animal disease control has also been tackled from another angle, that rather than seeking to alter the living conditions of the animals, instead seeks to alter the animals themselves. In this context, attempts have been made to rear strains of 'minimal-disease' animals which are kept in highly controlled environments (Webster 1994: 120). Poultry flocks today can be bred to be 'specific-pathogen free', which essentially means that particular disease-producing agents have been eliminated by breeding and rearing birds in sterile conditions. Such isolation, however, can render such birds vulnerable to other microorganisms that might otherwise have been innocuous (Mason and Singer 1980: 25–6).

Modern intensive livestock production is a risky business and sometimes it is human health that is at stake. In spite of the industry's endeavours to produce animal products that are safe for human consumption, as indicated above, food-borne infections still pose a threat to public health (Jones 1992: 107–36). The intensification of poultry rearing is the main culprit for bacterial infections in humans. Salmonella infection is one of the ever-present hazards of broiler rearing. It is in fact widely accepted that salmonella will persist in poultry stocks, although it can be kept at bay by good feeding and housing practices. The pervasiveness of this bacteria in poultry is largely due to contaminated feed, although people and wild animals or birds can also be the vectors of transmission (Brander and Ellis 1977: 12). Intensively reared poultry, like other farm animals which can carry the salmonella bacteria, are generally fed on high-protein feeds which can contain slaughterhouse waste and other animal by-products such as dried poultry manure. If such feed is inadequately sterilised, disease organisms can persist and can be passed on to other animals (Johnson 1991: 87). Sterilisation is a costly process which occurs through heat treatment. However, irradiation of animal feed is not always efficient because strains of salmonella have emerged which are heat-resistant and continue to contaminate feed (Schwabe 1984a).[3]

The transmission of salmonella requires 'the transfer of faeces or intestinal contents from an infected individual to the digestive tract of a susceptible one' (Schwabe 1984a: 552). Like animals, humans can become infected by salmonellosis through the ingestion of contaminated animal produce. The disease can cause gastroenteritis, septic shock syndrome and focal infection in humans, and can even be fatal to vulnerable individuals, such as infants or elderly people (Steele 1977). It should be emphasised that good hygiene and effective cooking methods from the abattoir to the kitchen can reduce the risk of infection for the human consumer. The modern systems of livestock rearing, mass animal transportation and conveyor belt style slaughterhouses, however, increase the possibilities of cross-infection and the contamination of human food. Although the most common bacterial infection, salmonella is not the only disease which may be contracted from the ingestion of animal produce. Bovine tuberculosis, brucellosis, trichinosis, campylobacteriosis, listeriosis, staphylococcal enterotoxicosis, clostridial toxicosis and toxoplasmosis may be transmitted through tainted animal food and cause human illness (Schwabe 1984a).[4]

Aside from food-borne infections and intoxications, consumer health is generally not affected by the diseases which farm animals carry. The people at greatest risk from agricultural animals and their products are in fact those who work with them; in other words, farm workers, veterinarians and individuals who handle animal carcasses occupationally. In western Europe today, the major zoonoses, such as brucellosis (contagious abortion), tuberculosis and anthrax, are uncommon. Other zoonotic diseases, however, present serious occupational hazards to those in the meat, dairy and animal product industry. For example, leptospirosis – commonly known as Weil's disease – is a disease which can seriously affect dairy farmers, both economically and physically. It is a contagious bacterial disease which can produce a high abortion rate in cattle late in pregnancy; it can be responsible for high mortality in calves, reduced milk production and contaminated milk. The organisms that cause leptospirosis are transmitted through urine and live in water or moist soil. Cattle – and other livestock – become infected through being splashed with infected urine, grazing on contaminated pasture or by drinking infected water. Other wild species, particularly rodents, are responsible for transmitting the disease to cattle, and humans can be infected by bathing in contaminated water or direct contact with infected urine (Blood 1994). The effect of leptospirosis on humans varies from inapparent to acute febrile illness which can be accompanied by fever, hepatitis, jaundice and meningitis – amongst other maladies (Schwabe 1986: 204). Good animal management, vaccination and reduction of contacts between livestock and rodents reduces the risks of infection by leptospirosis. There are many more health hazards for those who come into routine contact with food-producing animals. Other occupational hazards for humans are presented by rickettsial diseases, fungal infections (e.g. ringworm), chlamydia infections and respiratory viral diseases, in addition to bacterial infections such as those described above (Steele 1977; Schwabe 1984a).

The fact that intensive livestock production today happens within closed systems, away from public view, has much to do with the reduction of infection risks. Modern livestock housing is essentially designed to keep out disease-causing organisms and their vectors of transmission and to keep disease-free animals in. Such systems are far from foolproof; infection may, for example, occur through the drinking water or animal feed. Furthermore, farmers, stockmen and veterinarians may introduce disease to livestock. It is commonplace when one enters a livestock production unit for one to have to don special overalls and boots in order to minimise the possibility of introducing new pathogens to the animals from outside. However, keeping all visitors out, apart from stock and veterinary personnel, not only aids disease prevention and control, but to some extent prevents consumers from gaining a first-hand glimpse of the conditions under which their food is produced.[5]

Modern consumer society demands a continual, cheap and dependable supply of animal products which are pre-packaged and ready to enjoy: yet never before have the majority been so divorced from the production of the animal proteins which sustain them. The urban consumer is estranged from the origins of the food he eats and the leather he wears and has limited involvement in or knowledge of the circumstances of their production. The consumer is very much reliant on the producers and retailers to offer fresh and uncontaminated animal products – at a low price – on demand. The 'farm fresh' animal products which are nowadays found in urban supermarkets are however unlikely to have been produced locally, as was formerly the case. Animal produce may originate from farms and factories situated hundreds of kilometres from the consumer's domicile. The transport networks and storage capacities which today so efficiently ensure the swift despatch and delivery of farm-fresh animal produce to the consumer were not possible until recently.

Previously the movement of livestock and carcasses was fairly restricted, both within and across provincial or national borders, not only through lack of adequate transportation and refrigeration, but also due to the fear and possibility of the spread of contagious disease. As the previous chapter illustrated, once a sufficient level of understanding and knowledge of transmission and control through governmental intervention had been reached, disease could be better contained, cross-infection prevented and animals could be more safely moved from one location to another. Yet although governmental regulations pertaining to animal disease control have existed both nationally and internationally since last century, it is still possible for contaminated animals to slip the net and infect others (be they animal or human). Given that infected livestock or tissue can easily and quickly be moved from one (international) location to another, new opportunities for disease-producing organisms can develop in areas and amongst animal–human groups previously unaffected. The risk of disease can be further exacerbated by the failure to properly disinfect vehicles used for animal transportation, and delays in the transfer of live animals or meat from one place to another facilitate contagion further. Since, on an international level, animal movements are more likely to increase than decrease as a result of political and economic accord, the potential problem of animal disease transmission could, in the future, be one of increasing significance.

The intensification of the veterinary regime during the twentieth century

As the above discussion suggests, the possibilities for the transmission of infectious diseases are very real, most particularly given the risks posed by intensive systems of agricultural animal management and animal transportation. It is largely for this reason that veterinary medicine has become so important during the twentieth century in maintaining and monitoring animal health, to keep the spread of infectious disease in check and to ensure that farmers adhere to and understand the guidelines and regulations concerning disease prevention and control. Yet while disease *risks* may today be far greater than ever before, the danger of humans *actually* contracting diseases from contact with animals or the consumption of animal produce is in fact relatively small (Jones 1992).

Throughout the course of the twentieth century, the veterinary regime has continued to move from strength to strength. The state veterinary services that were instituted in the industrialised nations of Europe during the late nineteenth century have played an increasingly important role in the control and prevention of animal disease. Legislative measures to combat the effects, spread and introduction of contagious disease have been enforced with increasing vigour. The successes of earlier campaigns and stringent legal controls to stamp out the animal plagues that devastated European livestock populations provided the basis for future legislation. For example, as we saw in the previous chapter, veterinary inspection and the rigorous enforcement of all regulations pertaining to the importation, transport, sale, slaughter and destruction of livestock successfully led to the eradication of contagious bovine pleuropneumonia in the Netherlands by 1887 and Britain in 1898 (Kerstens 1971; MAFF 1965). The introduction of measures to financially compensate farmers for their losses through compulsory slaughter policies undoubtedly provided an incentive to abide by governmental regulations and allowed veterinary officials to perform their duties without hindrance. Eventual success in eradicating disease helped to persuade livestock producers to accept the ruthless and restrictive regulations that the state sought to enforce. As a consequence, state veterinary intervention has become institutionalised within modern livestock production. Moreover, during the twentieth century, the appreciation of the need for animal disease control and prevention has more or less been incorporated into the habitus of livestock producers.[6]

Scientific developments have, of course, played a crucial role in the prevention and control of animal disease. The development of the science of bacteriology, advances in pathology, parasitology, immunology and microbiology and so forth have provided important contributions to advances in animal and public health. By the turn of the century, European governments had become increasingly aware of the need for better scientific understanding of animal disease if they were to reduce the risks that it posed. In the Netherlands, for example, the State Serum Institute was founded in 1904 – by the pioneering veterinarian and bacteriologist Jan Poels – with a view to steering the work of the established Dutch

Veterinary Service towards more scientific means of preventing and curing livestock disease. The Serum Institute experimented with the production of a serum against foot-and-mouth disease and an anthrax vaccine. Moreover, it conducted bacteriological and chemical investigations into milk and dairy produce. Interestingly, this new institute operated specifically outside the dominion of the veterinary school, being instead an organ of the state (Offringa 1971: 234–5). In 1933, nearly three decades later, the State Veterinary Research Institute was established, primarily to study and develop a vaccine against foot-and-mouth disease – a highly infectious disease that has perhaps wreaked the greatest havoc on European livestock and the livestock industry during the twentieth century. By 1946, the Institute's director, H.S. Frenkel, had succeeded in developing a method by which a vaccine against foot-and-mouth disease could be produced in large quantities (Koolmees and Mathijsen 1993: 230). This method, however, only proved effective until 1951, when a more virulent strain of the disease struck Dutch livestock (Offringa 1981: 193).

From 1945 onwards, the structure of the state veterinary machine became increasingly more complex, as government-subsidised Animal Health Services were established in each province within the Netherlands. The earliest regional animal health service had in fact already been established in Friesland in 1919. Its early work led to significant progress in the battle against bovine tuberculosis. The new regional services were modelled on their Friesian predecessor and strove for the coordinated control of animal disease, involving not only scientific and governmental veterinary advisors, but also representatives of local farmers and dairy organisations and practising veterinarians. The eleven regional Animal Health Services were in turn coordinated by the Industrial Board for Agriculture, who established an Animal Health Committee to deal with the allocation of funds and organisation of schemes for disease control (Mol 1971: 43). After the Second World War, the regeneration of the meat and dairy export industry became an important part of Dutch economic recovery. A key aspect of this was a national plan to rid Dutch cattle herds of tuberculosis, thereby ensuring the safety and quality of the national product. A considerable portion of the Marshall Plan funds that were made available to the Netherlands to assist post-war economic reconstruction was devoted to achieve this end. By 1956, the disease had been conquered due to the efforts and cooperation of the Animal Health Services, practising veterinarians and the meat inspection service.

On the basis of this national plan's success, similarly successful attempts were made to control and eradicate brucellosis from the Dutch livestock population (Offringa 1981: 191–2).

By 1957, the Serum Institute and the State Veterinary Institute amalgamated to form the Central Veterinary Institute, which functioned under the auspices of the Dutch Ministry of Agriculture and Fisheries. The Veterinary Service was effectively given the governmental mandate, through the establishment of legislation such as the Livestock Act and the Veterinary Medicines Act, to prevent animal disease and preserve public health. The work of the Central Veterinary Institute continued to grow and diversify throughout the 1960s and 1970s. In 1986, it consolidated and moved to new premises in Lelystad (in the province of Flevoland). By 1994, the CVI amalgamated with a number of other agricultural animal research institutes to create the Institute for Animal Science and Health (ID-DLO 1995). Today, this institute employs over 600 people and conducts research into animal health, breeding and reproduction, animal welfare, stress and management, animal nutrition, and so forth. Moreover, it is responsible for diagnostic work, the production of vaccines, specific-pathogen free animals, diagnostic preparations, etc., and the control and standardisation of veterinary medicines.

The developments in state-directed animal disease control in the Netherlands can be mirrored in the rise of the State Veterinary Service in Great Britain. There too was an understanding for the necessity of improved scientific knowledge and diagnosis of animal disease. The first governmental diagnostic laboratory was set up in 1894 in response to an outbreak of swine fever. This was followed by the establishment of the Central Veterinary Laboratory at Weybridge, Surrey, in 1913. Initial research was conducted into spontaneous abortion, swine fever, scrapie, foot-and-mouth disease and diseases of poultry. As farmers began to increase the size of their flocks, as the process of intensification of production began to take off, the laboratory found itself increasingly dealing with the effects and greater incidence of poultry disease. During the 1930s, the laboratory began to research and produce tuberculin, in addition to an anti-abortion vaccine (MAFF 1965: 311–12). The Agricultural Act of 1937 facilitated further expansion of the laboratory. New research departments of bacteriology, biochemistry, parasitology, pathology and poultry disease were established and a further laboratory was set up in Scotland (Dunlop and Williams 1996: 556).

By 1960, the Animal Health Division successfully completed its programme to eradicate tuberculosis from the British cattle population. During the 1960s, the new challenges to animal health presented by the changing methods in livestock production gave extra impetus to the fight against animal disease. The intensive rearing of calves, for example, led to an increasing incidence of respiratory disease. This unforeseen consequence of new methods of animal husbandry required urgent bacteriological and virological investigation (MAFF 1965: 315). Similarly, the development of artificial insemination and its widespread use in cattle presented new problems for animal disease control. The movement of inseminators between farms and the importation of and trade in semen presented new hazards for the transmission of infectious animal disease. In 1955, legislative measures were taken to prohibit importation of foreign animal semen without a licence and the Animal Health Division took steps to screen the health of bulls (MAFF 1965: 295).

In addition to the Central Veterinary Laboratory, the Veterinary Investigation Service was established in 1922, with regional centres throughout Britain. This service essentially provided local laboratory facilities on which practising veterinarians could rely to help diagnose and investigate animal health problems in the herds that they attended (MAFF 1965: 329). Initially, the Veterinary Investigation Centres were attached to agricultural colleges, but in 1946 they were incorporated into the Ministry of Agriculture, Fisheries and Food. The interaction between local veterinarians, veterinary investigation officers, the researchers of the Central Veterinary Laboratory and legislators in fact provides a good illustration of the increasing complexity of animal disease control during the twentieth century. At the grassroots level, practising veterinary surgeons observe and report the local incidence of animal disease. This in turn is investigated by veterinary investigation officers who conduct field investigations and epidemiological studies to gauge the extent of animal health problems. In the meantime, the Central Veterinary Laboratory attempts to understand the aetiology of the disease and explores how it may effectively be controlled. These combined investigations may in turn lead to the inception of statutory control measures, vaccination, test and slaughter programmes to contain and eradicate animal disease. In Britain, this kind of cooperation eventually led to the eradication of brucellosis and is today responsible for the investigation and extensive monitoring of new pathogens and diseases, e.g. bovine spongiform encephalopathy. In October 1995, the Central Veterinary

Laboratory and the Veterinary Investigation Service merged to form the Veterinary Laboratories Agency in a further bid to improve the collaboration necessary to ensure animal disease control and the provision of advice to the Ministry of Agriculture, Fisheries and Food and other veterinary health workers (CVL 1994).

Throughout the twentieth century, the necessity for collaboration and cooperation has extended far beyond the activities of local and nationally organised veterinary organisations. As illustrated in the previous chapter, international cooperation on matters of veterinary public health first began during the nineteenth century as a result of the devastation caused by the cattle plague. In 1924, the *Office International des Epizooties* was established in Paris. This intergovernmental organisation initially sought to promote and coordinate research into the control and surveillance of animal disease, and has remained active on this front to this day; its original membership of 28 having gradually been expanded to some 144 member states. During the post-war period, additional international fora for dealing with the economic and health problems associated with animal disease were institutionalised. In Europe, the European Union – and its former incarnations, i.e. the EEC and EC – have provided the main political arena within which European governments can jointly discuss and legislate on matters pertaining to veterinary public health and animal welfare. The European Economic Community (EEC) was originally established in 1958 – following the signing of the Treaties of Rome (1957) – with a view to achieving economic and political union amongst its member states, namely Belgium, Germany, France, Italy, Luxembourg and the Netherlands. In 1973, Denmark, Great Britain and Ireland became members of the EEC. In later years, Austria, Greece, Finland, Spain, Sweden and Portugal joined the ranks of states seeking European economic union; the organisation is set to expand yet further in future as former Eastern Bloc countries vie for membership.

Since its inception, the European Union has had a critical impact on agricultural practice and the trade in live animals and animal produce within Europe. The Common Agricultural Policy was instituted during the early 1960s with a view to increasing agricultural productivity, ensuring a fair standard of living for the agricultural community, stabilising markets, ensuring food supplies and providing consumers with food at reasonable prices. It has been perhaps the most important Common Policy that operates within the Union and has served as an important precursor to the 'single market' that is today intended to guarantee the free movement of goods, services, capital and people between the fifteen member states. The Common Agricultural Policy greatly influenced the economics of livestock farming within Europe and initially encouraged farmers to intensify production. Ultimately this led to massive overproduction and the creation of huge surpluses, which in turn depressed market prices. 'Butter and beef mountains' came to symbolise the crisis in European agriculture; livestock numbers needed to be reduced and milk quotas were introduced. The Common Agricultural Policy has consequently undergone significant reforms and today it even encourages the *extensification* of production methods, particularly in the beef sector.

Free trade between member states remains at the top of the European Union's agenda, and trade naturally includes the trade in livestock and animal produce. As the epizootics of the past clearly evidenced, the movement of animals across national borders presents potentially great hazards to both public and animal health. Each member state has its own internal legislation and procedures regarding the control and prevention of livestock disease; the efficacy of which is entirely dependent on the efficiency of and cooperation between livestock producers, veterinarians and governmental agencies. However, membership of the European Union has required that each country's system of animal disease control be brought in line with those of other member states, in order to ensure a harmonisation and uniformity of disease prevention. Moreover, a system of veterinary inspection and veterinary and livestock regulations have necessarily been introduced in an attempt to ensure the health of animals and the safety of meat that are crossing national borders.

With regard to livestock, each animal that is traded between member states, or enters the Union from a non-member state, must be accompanied by a veterinary health certificate that has been signed by an official veterinarian. Two types of certificates exist: one for animals intended for breeding and production; and another for animals intended for slaughter. The health requirements for breeding animals are much more stringent than for those destined for slaughter. These certificates detail the animal's origins, destination, means of transport, age, breed, type, means of identification and whether they passed through a market or assembly point. Such certificates are valid for ten days after the animal has been loaded for transport. In this way, diseased animals can be traced along with those that they came into contact with during transport. The health certificate states that the animal has been examined and has been passed as healthy by an official veterinarian and that it originates from a herd or region free from specified diseases. Animals may have to undergo further tests depending on their origin, type and destination. Traded livestock must meet a number of welfare considerations determined on a Union-wide basis. Likewise, the rules for the trade in meat have been harmonised throughout the European Union, in order that animal flesh is produced, preserved and transported according to rules of hygiene identical to every member state. Certificates issued by official veterinarians at the place of meat production provide a guarantee that the meat is fit for consumption and serve as a valid transport document which testifies to the safety of the product. Produce from outside the European Union is subject to similar checks at border inspection posts and is required to meet the standards deemed acceptable within the Union (Veenman 1995–7).

The veterinary regime has thus been further consolidated on an international level and has led – at least in principle – to the standardisation of the control of animal disease, welfare and healthcare and the quality of meat and other foods of animal origin within Europe. The legislators in Brussels have ensured that member states adopt uniform policies with regard to livestock production. European legislation, therefore, has increasingly come to determine the nature of national legislation. For example, since 1988, EU countries have maintained a ban on all growth-stimulating hormones, although such products are still widely employed in the USA (Johnson 1991: 76–7). Attempts to eliminate the illegal trade in such hormone products even led to the murder of a Belgian veterinary inspector in 1995. An illustration of the impact of the EU's veterinary regulations on member states can also be provided by events surrounding the bovine spongiform encephalopathy (BSE) crisis. The severity of the legislation has greatly disabled the British livestock and meat trade and has also had significant repercussions for other countries. It seems likely that the public health issues and trade problems surrounding BSE will continue to feature prominently on the European economic, agricultural and veterinary agenda in Brussels in the future. Similarly, the way the 1997 outbreak of classical swine fever in the Netherlands has been dealt with has to a great extent been affected by EU regulations. While vaccination may provide the key to ending the crisis, the EU has committed itself to a policy of eradication of classical swine fever and, at present, forbids the use of a vaccine which may be effective against the disease. The Dutch pig industry has been crippled by this outbreak, export embargoes have been instituted and over three million pigs have been destroyed, not necessarily because they had contracted the disease, but to prevent overcrowding of pig stalls.

While animal disease control and prevention measures have become increasingly stringent throughout Europe during the twentieth century, leading to the virtual eradication of the majority of animal plagues that decimated livestock and played havoc with the European economy in centuries past, we cannot forget that the modern global economy and the routine movement of individuals – both human and animal – across and between continents also have a bearing on veterinary public health within the bounds of Europe. Diseases such as tuberculosis and classical swine fever, for example, are known to have been transmitted to western European livestock from live animal imports or animal produce from eastern Europe. Similarly, imports from countries where animal disease control is not so advanced or strict may still pose a threat to public health since spores of diseases such as anthrax, which have more or less been eradicated in advanced Western societies, can still be introduced through the import of hides, animal foods etc. from regions where the disease still persists.[7] It must also be noted that while a highly effective veterinary regime exists within Europe, veterinary policing is not always as efficient as it should be and regulations are not always well enforced. Essentially, it only takes one weak link in the chain of interdependencies involved in the process of transforming animals into safe food to lead to inefficiencies and failures in animal disease control. Again, the recent BSE crisis provides a clear example of this. Inadequate compliance with and policing of the meat and bone meal bans, first introduced by the British government in 1988 to prevent the feeding of mammalian protein to ruminants, appear to have allowed the epidemic to continue, when it might otherwise have been curtailed. One may thus conclude that any animal disease control measures that the legislators introduce can only be as good as their policing.

The control of animal disease today is far from simply a local or regional problem, it has instead become a global one. The involvement of veterinary experts in the policy making and execution of the World Health Organisation (WHO) and the Food and Agriculture Organisation (FAO) certainly attests to this. However, although advanced industrialised societies have the animal disease problem more or less under control – producing significant animal protein surpluses in spite of continuing population growth – the (rural) populations of developing nations across the globe continue to suffer both the economic and health effects of animal disease. Furthermore, animal diseases can affect livestock populations and food production to such an extent that they do not even return a profit (Steele 1977). Livestock disease therefore not only generates economic problems, but also wastes resources which could help to solve the problem of world food shortages.[8]

While the focus of this chapter is far from global, it is still important to be aware of the fact that the relationship between humans, animals and the environment in which they all live is a continually changing one which is not confined within national borders. The complexity and scale of interdependencies between humans and other animals is such today that failure to keep disease-causing microorganisms adequately in check could be potentially devastating for both the physical and economic health of world populations. The necessity of an effective and globally-oriented veterinary regime in present-day society is, therefore, manifest.

The role of the modern large-animal practitioner

Thus far, this chapter has largely concentrated on the veterinary regime as enforced by the state within an international arena. Scant attention has yet been paid to the role of the individual veterinary surgeon who is responsible for the everyday veterinary care and treatment of livestock. Throughout this century, the veterinarian's role has changed quite dramatically from treating individual animals to the management of herd-health. This shift from curative to preventative veterinary medicine began to take place during the early 1960s. Until the early twentieth century, the veterinary profession had directed itself largely to the care and treatment of horses and the study of equine disease. The invention of the internal combustion engine, however, led to a rapid decline in the importance of horses within European society. Work horses and pit ponies were put out to pasture or sent to the knacker's yard as motorised vehicles were introduced to do their work. Horses declined in military importance as new technologies were introduced. This century thus bore witness to the last major conflicts fought on horseback, ending centuries of equine dominance in warfare. Military horses are now maintained almost solely for ceremonial purposes. During the twentieth century, the noble mount has largely been relegated to the realms of pleasure and sport. Even the veterinary surgeon eventually abandoned his trusty steed for the automobile to make his daily rounds. Today, the veterinarian's car functions almost as a veterinary surgery on wheels; stocked with every conceivable medicine and surgical instrument that he may need to treat his animal patients, in addition to a mobile telephone.

As the importance of horses and equine medicine declined, the veterinary profession shifted its focus to food-producing animals; the health of which had been growing in veterinary importance since the late nineteenth century due to the new scientific understanding of the relationship between animal disease and public health. Meat inspection, for example, became a new arena for veterinary expertise and responsibility during the early 1900s (Koolmees 1997). In addition to this, as we shall see in the following chapter, the ever-increasing popularity of pet-keeping opened up new avenues and markets for the veterinary profession, leading to specialisation and a massive expansion in small-animal practice: this development will be discussed in the following chapter. The face of everyday veterinary practice has continued to change as antibiotics, vaccines, anaesthetics and analgesics have been introduced to aid the treatment and cure of animal patients. Likewise, improved surgical instrumentation and equipment to facilitate operations and diagnosis – e.g. restraining devices, operating tables, X-ray machines etc. – have transformed the conditions and effectiveness of veterinary work (Dunlop and Williams 1996: 659–60).

Furthermore, the call for veterinary education has greatly increased throughout the twentieth century. The veterinary schools that were founded during the late eighteenth and early nineteenth centuries have continued to expand and diversify, attracting increasingly more students, including – for the first time – women, who today constitute a substantial percentage of veterinary school (under)graduates. The veterinary curriculum has been transformed in line with the shifting interest from equine medicine to the diseases and health of food-producing animals and, certainly after the Second World War, pets. Further to this, the scientific, technological and pharmaceutical developments of the twentieth century have greatly influenced the nature and content of veterinary education, as has the ever-increasing importance of veterinary public health to society. Today, veterinary students receive instruction in the fields of veterinary anatomy, physiology, pathology, microbiology, parasitology, animal husbandry and reproduction, pharmacology and pharmacotherapy, immunology, radiology, biomolecular science, food hygiene and animal nutrition, in addition to being trained in veterinary surgery and given clinical instruction in specialities such as obstetrics and anaesthesiology. Graduates are not necessarily destined to become practising veterinary surgeons, they may instead elect to pursue a career in public service (e.g. meat inspection), or find gainful employment within the private sector, for example, in the pharmaceutical or animal feed industry. Alternatively, the veterinary graduate may, for instance, end up working in the field of laboratory animal science, or may specialise in the treatment of wild or zoo animals. Nevertheless, whatever the course the veterinary graduate's career may take, he or she will have received a training which will qualify him or her to treat agricultural, recreational and pet animals, in addition to having been educated in veterinary public health.

Veterinarians are thus engaged in a broad spectrum of activities involving animals, ranging from the treatment of domesticated animals, both large and small, to food inspection, wild animal medicine, laboratory animal science, veterinary pharmaceutics and public health management. Yet although the tasks of veterinary professionals may be so very disparate, they are actually all part and parcel of a single profession that is governed by – at least on a national level – a central professional body that sets down the code of ethics and professional conduct to which all veterinarians are expected to adhere. However, despite the great diversity that exists within the profession, the fact remains that when one thinks of veterinarians, one generally conjures images of Herriotesque animal doctors who rescue and care for sick and injured pets or farm animals. Such veterinarians, i.e. small- and large-animal practitioners, have indeed been the focus of this study, but – as I quickly discovered early on in my research – they do not and cannot always live up to the romantic paragons of fiction. To understand the nature of veterinary work, one must forget the popular image of the intrepid animal doctor, battling to save the lives of sick and injured animals. Although veterinary heroics such as patching up accident victims and helping animals in labour are a constituent – and the most fulfilling part – of their work, veterinarians spend most of their time performing extremely routine and unheroic deeds. In reality, veterinarians are endlessly preoccupied with performing highly routine procedures pertaining to the management, control and prevention of disease and parasitic infection. Unlike their predecessors, modern veterinarians are involved more with the surveillance of herd-health than the treatment of individual patients. For example, it is now standard for poultry to be treated as a flock, rather than be examined individually. Large-animal practitioners are required to spend an inordinate amount of time engaged in taking blood samples for analysis by governmental agencies and inoculating livestock herds en masse against a wide variety of infectious diseases which may otherwise impede production and the livestock and meat trade. Likewise, the small-animal practitioner is preoccupied with vaccinating the pet animal population. The bulk of routine veterinary work is thus preventative, rather than curative. It is aimed at preserving animal resources, to keep animals fit and healthy in order that they may efficiently service human needs, whatever those needs may be. Ultimately the veterinarian's role today is to help farmers maintain healthy, disease-free animals and to prevent the spread of diseases to other livestock or humans; the animal healing with which one generally associates the veterinary profession is in many ways secondary to this task.

The practising veterinary surgeon is, therefore, one of the most important cogs in the wheels of the complex machinery that is responsible for the transformation of living flesh into animal produce fit for human consumption. Before animals ever reach the slaughterhouse, the herds or flocks from which they originate will have been closely monitored by local veterinarians who, on behalf of the regional governmental animal health service, collect blood samples from individual animals or entire herds in order to detect, or rule out the possibility of, infection. The elaborate system of individual livestock registration and ear-tagging that exists today has greatly improved the precision of this process.[9] Vets will generally receive their instructions to visit specific farms and take blood samples from a given number of animals. They are provided with sheets of labels on which the bar-codes of individual animals are printed. It is then simply a task of going to the farm, matching the bar-codes to individual animals, tapping blood into test-tubes, sticking the appropriate labels on the tubes and sending them to the laboratory for analysis. This is the kind of laborious task with which veterinarians today are generally preoccupied, which also involves a substantial amount of paperwork to deal with the governmental bureaucracy related to disease prevention. Mandatory visits to farms to tap blood from or vaccinate animals can, however, provide a veterinarian with the opportunity to inspect a herd and identify health problems without him necessarily having been called out by the farmer for any specific purpose.

Prior to slaughter, animals are again required to be inspected by a veterinarian. There will also be a post-mortem inspection of the animals to ensure their suitability for human consumption. In short, before it gets anywhere near the human consumer, animal tissue is supposed to be free of disease, not to mention various veterinary drug residues which could be passed into the food chain.[10] Similarly, milk from dairy herds is routinely checked for evidence of brucellosis, tuberculosis and mastitis so that it will be safe for human consumption. This testing for disease organisms is, of course, in addition to the hygienic milking practices, sterile bottling of milk and obligatory pasteurisation which have been deemed necessary to bring clean and safe milk products into consumers' homes. The strict veterinary control and inspection of agricultural animals generally means that domestic animal products are highly unlikely to be of any great hazard to consumers; though, as periodic outbreaks of salmonellosis confirm, disease control measures, while better than in the past, are still far from infallible.[11] Today, the people who are most likely to contract zoonotic diseases are veterinarians or farm workers, rather than the general public.

Apart from disease control, the management of animal reproduction is a task still situated high up on the everyday veterinary agenda. The veterinarian plays an important role in the control of the size of animal populations and overseeing the (re)production of healthy and efficient animals. This work includes neutering pet animals and providing obstetric and post-natal care for animals. Further to this, the veterinarian is entrusted the task of, what can best be described as, 'routine animal maintenance'. In other words, they are involved in the repair, rehabilitation or destruction of sick and injured animals. Non-therapeutic surgical interventions, such as dehorning, tail-docking, etc., to facilitate livestock management and control animal behaviour – or to accommodate the aesthetic whims of pet owners – are also routinely performed by veterinarians. The veterinarian will treat dermatological conditions, advise on appropriate animal care, nutrition and housing, attend to dental problems and other matters relating to animal health and welfare. Veterinarians are, therefore, charged with the overall responsibility of helping animal owners maintain an abundant and healthy animal population. They thus play a crucial, though much overlooked, social role by maintaining the animal resources on which human society depends and ensuring the perpetuation of the veterinary regime.

6

PANDERING TO PETS

Pet-keeping and the emergence of small-animal practice

Introduction

Although the relationship between humans and other animals has changed radically throughout the course of human history, it is during the twentieth century that the most profound changes in the relationship between humans and domesticated animals have occurred. As the previous chapter clearly illustrated, this century has borne witness to the exploitation of animal resources on a scale far grander than ever before. Most striking is how the cleft between ourselves and food-producing animals has grown as these animals have increasingly been accorded the status of machines through the development of the intensive farming practices that have been deemed necessary to meet ever-growing human food demands. Yet while the divide between ourselves and food-producing animals clearly continues to expand, our identification with and dependence on the smaller, and more cuddly, species which we keep as pets has also grown. It often seems that we increasingly keep pets to satisfy our emotional, rather than material, needs and gain tactile comfort and trust from them which might not be found elsewhere in our modern lives.

This penultimate chapter is devoted to our relationship with small domesticated animals and will explore how the veterinary regime has been extended to the treatment and care of such animals and their diseases. Our relationship with pet animals stands in sharp contrast to the agricultural animals that have thus far been discussed. Cattle, horses, sheep, goats, pigs and poultry have always played a clearly defined role within human society as the providers of food, raw materials and muscle power, whereas dogs and cats have generally been of limited economic utility and nutritional value. The way in which small animals have been treated – both culturally and medically – is, however, illustrative of the ever-changing and eternally ambiguous nature of human–animal relations. Moreover, our increasing concern for the health and welfare of small animals further manifests how the dual processes of expansion and specialisation have affected and led to intensification of the veterinary regime during the twentieth century. Again, as in preceding chapters, the theme of the relationship between animal disease and public health will be returned to. In this regard, I shall consider the ways in which our increasingly close associations with small animal species have either benefited human health, or alternatively posed a potential threat to it. First, however, I will briefly examine humankind's apparently universal proclivity for keeping small animals as pets, in addition to exploring the increasing popularity of pet-keeping throughout human history.

Why do we keep small animals as pets?

The human penchant for keeping animals as pets is certainly a most curious one. It is a practice that is apparently universal in nature and most likely pre-dates the inception of livestock keeping and animal husbandry. The earliest evidence of an association between human and animal based on affection rather than gastronomy dates back some 12,000 years. In 1977, a Natufian tomb, discovered in northern Israel, was found to contain the remains of an elderly human whose hand appears to have been deliberately placed on the skeleton of a wolf/dog puppy. From this archaeologists have deduced the probable existence of an affectionate bond in life between the two (Davis 1987: 145–8). Further to this, as discussed earlier in Chapter 2, anthropological and historical observations of pet-keeping in hunter-gatherer societies have provided the basis for speculation on the existence and nature of pet-keeping in early human societies. Just why humans have shown such a universal proclivity for keeping small animals as pets has been the source of considerable debate. Yi-Fu Tuan (1984), for example, has suggested that pet-keeping stemmed from humankind's insecurity and trepidation of the natural world which has led to an innate desire and need to gain control over and subdue nature. Keeping pets could, in this way, be viewed as a means of 'playfully' exercising human ascendancy over the natural world. Perhaps this psychological impulse to control may well have provided a basis for the apparently ubiquitous practice of pet-keeping, but there are a whole host of other explanations that might more concretely explain the age-old appeal of keeping animals, particularly dogs and cats, as pets.

Dogs and cats are in fact the two species that have most successfully and persistently appealed to human affections throughout history and, as a result, are today the most common species kept as household pets. There are a number of fairly obvious reasons why people seem to always have appreciated having such animals around. First, from early times, dogs were valued for their ability to help track and detect game, and later to help herd other domesticated animals rather than prey on them. Likewise, cats were easily tolerated since their natural talent for vermin control helped to protect precious grain supplies. A second plausible reason for the widespread appeal and practice of keeping dogs and cats is that, more than any other, these two species appear to have been able to fit into human social organisation more readily than any other kinds of animal. Both dogs and cats are inherently social animals that are able, at least when exposed to humans from an early age, to form relationships with humans. Moreover, since they do not have to be caged, they – often by nature – remain attached to the people with whom and the locations where they live. Thirdly, these animals have been quite readily kept around human households because they are quite easy to maintain and house-train. Furthermore, apart from a few (artificially engineered) breeds of dog, their size and strength are generally not threatening to humans, either adult or child, and yet they are large enough for humans to be able to relate to them as individual personalities. The relatively high intelligence of these species and their playfulness have added greatly to their appeal. A fourth possible explanation for their popularity as pets is that people seem to find it particularly easy to anthropomorphise cats and dogs, for both species are particularly communicative and possess an extensive range of facial expressions, typical body and tail postures, sounds and so forth that humans believe they can understand (CSS report 1988: 8). As a corollary to this, it has been suggested that canines use their facial muscles in a very similar way to primates to express emotion: this could perhaps account for the success of canine communication with humans (Messent and Serpell 1981: 14). Finally, the life-span of dogs and cats tends to be quite long in comparison with other small animals, thus providing greater opportunities for strong and sometimes deep relationships to develop between animal and owner.

It is interesting that there is an apparent preference to acquire such animals as pets when they are still in infancy. There has been a great deal of speculation as to the reasons why baby animals are particularly attractive to humans. It has, for example, been suggested that infant animals – with their soft fluffy fur and huge eyes – provoke a 'cute response' in humans and, with these infantile qualities they appeal to and evoke a 'strong desire to nurture and provide parental care and affection' (Serpell 1996: 83). As helpless infants, frequently taken from their mothers too young, they are entirely dependent on humans for their survival and remain so throughout their entire lives. They thus in a sense retain their childlike qualities and, it appears, can be treated and talked to by their owners as if they were real children. This penchant for baby animals has also been reflected in the domestication process as animals, particularly dogs, have been specifically bred to appeal to human sentiments. Attractive and paedomorphic physiological and behavioural traits have often been favoured, leading to the creation of many miniature breeds that appear to retain an infantile character and appearance throughout adulthood; this is also known as neoteny (Serpell 1996; Voith 1981). The terms 'lap' and 'toy' reflect the clearly intended function of these dogs. Along with their size, these dogs are often bred so that their eyes are protuberant and large, their noses squashed and jaws foreshortened to appeal, perhaps comically, to humans to attain a cute response (Serpell 1996: 82–3). While these breeds might well be more attractive to humans, their features are nothing more than physical defects that can handicap the animals and cause them considerable pain. In recent years, irresponsible (inter)breeding to meet, or exceed, fashionable breeding standards has very much compromised animal welfare by causing and perpetuating such hereditary defects.

One of the main questions that any discussion on pet-keeping inevitably raises is whether people are motivated to keep pets as substitutes for human contact and relationships. Dogs and cats have played an increasingly important role in modern industrial society. It has, for example, been estimated that approximately 50 per cent of all households within the European Union keep animals as pets (Endenburg 1991: 13). Many explanations of pet-keeping link the growing popularity of this practice to urbanisation, loss of ties and contact with others, decline in birth rates and family size, and so forth. However, while such explanations are convincing, they fail to adequately address the issue of whether animals are acquired as pets to meet a human need or desire to create, or have, a loving relationship with a significant other in the absence of the 'real thing', i.e. another human. It is fair to say that animals are sometimes treated as a kind of 'transitional object' (Winnicott 1980): people may project human-style friendship and personality onto other creatures through anthropomorphism especially, it seems, when they have little or no contact with others. Occasionally, this can be taken to extremes and the relationship between person and pet can become sexual or pathological in nature.

Nevertheless, suggesting that pets are by their very nature living transitional objects is highly over-simplistic, for it fails to take into account the fact that such animals fulfil very diverse functions in human social life apart from companionship. Although it is a very significant function of pet-keeping, companionship is not always the prime motive or reason for acquiring and keeping an animal as a pet. Moreover, when one considers that pet-keeping is today even more popular amongst people who cohabit or have families than single and elderly people – in other words, its popularity is greatest among people with normal and regular social and emotional contacts – it becomes clear that pets are perhaps significant to humans quite independently of, or maybe additionally to, providing an emotional crutch in the absence of meaningful relationships with other human beings (Endenburg 1991). Rather than providing substitutes for human contacts, pets may, in fact offer a kind of relationship that human–human contact does not, or rarely, provide. The fact that a pet is not human and lacks human foibles may equally add to its attraction and provide motivation for acquiring one. In the following, I shall delve a little deeper into the nature of the human–pet relationship, by unearthing the historical roots of pet-keeping and briefly examining the great diversity in our attitudes towards and treatment of small animals throughout the ages.

A brief history of pet-keeping

As the above discussion has already suggested, the practice of keeping small animals as pets is a ubiquitous one that can be traced back to well before the existence of written records. Yet although it is clear that an affectionate bond has long existed between human and animal, it does not necessarily follow that such warmth towards animals has always been shared by all. In fact, quite to the contrary, as we shall shortly see, the practice of pet-keeping has been ridiculed or reviled and small animals have been subject to all manner of abuse at the hands of their human masters. It must not be forgotten that the animals that we have commonly kept as pets have also served other social and utilitarian functions throughout history: they have, for example, served as beasts of burden, protectors of property, partners in hunting, religious icons and agents of pest control, not to mention being the subjects of scientific experimentation and sporting amusement. Even today, within modern western society, where pet animals are kept in greater numbers and held in higher esteem than ever before, there exists a great deal of ambiguity and ambivalence with regard to our interactions with small domesticates. Thus, while it is true to say that dogs and cats can be cherished as pets, it is also the case that these animals may be severely maltreated and abandoned by their owners, or even employed for – what many may today consider barbarous – sporting or scientific ends. We must, therefore, exercise great care in making sweeping statements about the human–pet animal relationship: one dog owner may dote on his dachshund, another may beat it to death. It is largely for this reason that I have avoided using the popular term 'companion animal' in this book. In my view, this term can be far from appropriate in describing the role and status of small animals in human society both past and present.

It has often been assumed that pet-keeping in centuries past was always the sole preserve of the rich; a trivial and luxurious practice that was the pure product of material affluence. Most certainly the various social elites – both aristocratic and ecclesiastical – who have wielded their power over the impoverished masses throughout history have distinguished themselves by their remarkable fondness for keeping animals of apparently no utilitarian function. However, this is not to say that the peasantry and the lower classes of the past were completely immune to the practice. As James Serpell has pointed out, the main victims of the English witch trials of the late sixteenth and seventeenth centuries, who were condemned partly on the basis that they possessed and showed affection for small animals – thought to be their demonic familiars – were generally poverty-stricken and elderly people (Serpell 1987 and 1996). Nonetheless, the vast majority of small animals that were kept by the masses were most likely owned for purely utilitarian purposes. Not that this necessarily precluded the existence of a close attachment between animal and owner; sheepdogs, in particular, have since antiquity often been held in considerable esteem. But, as Keith Thomas – writing on working dogs during the seventeenth century – observes, even dogs valued for their practical functions were frequently disposed of in an unpleasant manner, once they had 'outlived their usefulness' (Thomas 1983: 102).

Unfortunately, the historical record of pet-keeping in European society derives most of its detail from the antics and peculiarities of the ruling elites and the well-to-do, rather than from the activities of the rank and file. Yet even there, the profoundly ambiguous nature of our relationship with small animals can be clearly discerned. Accounts of pet-keeping throughout the ages have consistently revealed the contempt felt towards those who made a habit of doting on, what were regarded as, essentially 'useless' animals. Lap-dogs, in particular, have always fallen foul to perhaps the most scathing criticism. In ancient Greece, for example, the keeping of such animals was keenly satirised by authors such as Theophrastus and Lucian (Serpell 1996: 46–7). From the late middle ages onwards, the practice of keeping 'toy' dogs became increasingly fashionable within aristocratic circles. While nobles and gentlemen held their hunting hounds and coursing dogs in the greatest esteem, their lady-folk cherished their smaller canine companions with similar intensity. Mediaeval noble women, for example, were inclined to carry such dogs around with them and feed them with scraps from the table, much to the disgruntlement of contemporary experts in etiquette (Serpell 1996: 49; Thomas 1983: 104). By the sixteenth century, the practice of keeping lap-dogs had become extremely popular within English high society, leading John Caius – a learned contemporary author on the subject of all things canine – to comment somewhat acrimoniously on the female penchant for keeping such dogs by writing that

> These dogges are litle, pretty, proper, and fyne, and sought for to satisfie the delicatenesse of daintie dames, and wanton womens wills, instrumentes of folly for them to play and dally withall, to tryfle away the treasures of time, to withdraw their mindes from more commendable exercises, and to content their corrupted concupiscences with vaine disport. (A selly shift to shunne yrksome ydlnesse.) These puppies the smaller they be, the more pleasure they preuoke, to more meete play fellowes for minsing mistresses to bear in their bosoms, to keepe company withal in their chambers, to succour with sleep in bed, and nourishe with meat at bourde, to lay in their lappes, and licke their lippes as they ryde in their waggons, and for good reason it should be so, for coursenesse with fynesse hath no fellowship, but featness with neatnesse hath neighbourhood enough. That plausible prouerbe verified vpon a Tyraunt, namely that he loued his sow better than his

> sonne, may well be applied to these kinde of people, who delight more in dogges that are depriued of all possibility of reason, then they doe in children that be capeable of wisedom and iudgement. But this abuse peraduenture raigneth where there hath bene long lacke of issue, or else where barrennes is the best blossome of bewty.
>
> (Caius 1576: 20–1)

Caius' accusation, that such women had a tendency to care more for their dogs than their children, was a common one. Thomas (1983: 108) similarly recounts that the preachers of this era were apt to bemoan the fact that fashionable women were known to neglect their own offspring in favour of their pet dogs. Likewise, it was remarked that the aristocracy treated their hunting hounds far better than they did their own human servants (Thomas ibid.: 103–4). This bent for holding small animals in higher regard than fellow human beings was, however, not the sole preserve of the wealthy members of sixteenth- and seventeenth-century English society. As James Serpell has observed, from ancient times up until the present day, members of the ruling elite have lavished their pet animals with affection, while concurrently displaying complete indifference to the plight of the impoverished masses. It is for this reason, he argues, that pet-keeping has become an extremely potent symbol of 'man's inhumanity to man' (Serpell 1996: 55).

By the sixteenth and seventeenth centuries, the practice of keeping pet animals had gradually begun to filter down from the very highest echelons of society to the households of the middle class, particularly those living in towns; pets thus became a permanent fixture in many ordinary urban homes (Thomas 1983: 110). The increasing urban population was in fact to play a key role in both the future spread of pet-keeping and changing attitudes towards animals. During the late eighteenth century, the face of European society began to change quite radically as the dual processes of industrialisation and urbanisation got under way. Commerce and manufacturing rapidly overtook agriculture as the primary source of wealth, causing mass migration to urban areas. As suggested in Chapter 4, it was at this time that new sensibilities towards animals slowly began to emerge. Diminishing contact with animals essentially meant that the urban population became far removed from the harsh realities of the human–animal relationship and were less inclined to regard animals in a purely utilitarian fashion. This development coincided with the more general changes in the personality structure of individuals that have been described by Norbert Elias in *The Civilising Process* (1994). Within this new emotional climate, there was an increasing latitude for sentimentality towards animals, and pets provided the ideal outlet for it to be expressed.

It has been suggested that pet-keeping only emerged as a widespread phenomenon once people had begun to gain a far greater mastery over the natural world. Harriet Ritvo (1987a, b), for example, has contended that it was the scientific, technological and economic developments of the late eighteenth and nineteenth centuries that made nature inherently less threatening and far more manageable; people, at least those living in urban areas, were no longer involved in a daily struggle with the forces of nature in order to survive. Yet while divorced from nature, she argues, pet-keeping at the same time provided a concrete link to it; keeping animals as pets clearly exemplified humankind's domination over the natural world. To support this claim, Ritvo discusses the enterprise of dog breeding during this period, arguing that the whole business of maintaining and improving existing breeds was a 'metaphorical assertion of domination'. Breeders increasingly played God in their attempts to produce increasing varieties and to control animal reproduction. Even those canine breeds, such as the collie, that had formerly performed a specific utilitarian function were aesthetically reconstructed according to the whims and desires of this new breed of dog fanciers. Kennel clubs, dog breeding associations and the practice of 'showing' pedigree animals emerged from the mid-nineteenth century onwards to service this growing passion for producing tailor-made animals (Ritvo 1987b: 161–3).

Until this time, dog breeds had developed largely in geographical isolation, according to the environment in which they lived and the manner in which they had been moulded to fulfil different functions for humans. Dog breeding had been the occupation of the aristocracy who sought in general to produce dogs that were suitable to assist every aspect of hunting, e.g. for the retrieval of birds, hare coursing, etc. As the Orient and the New World became more accessible, new breeds were introduced and kept by the wealthy as pets. By the nineteenth century, for example, toy Chinese dogs had come to replace the toy spaniels and pugs that had enjoyed popularity as lap-dogs during the sixteenth and seventeenth centuries respectively (Thomas 1983: 107). From the nineteenth century onwards, both the spread of pet-keeping to all levels of society and the development of a greater understanding of eugenics and cynology, led to the increasing diversification of breeds. As a consequence of this artificial selection and the genetic malleability of the species, an adult dog today can weigh between two and eighty kilos; this being in contrast to the wolf, the closest wild species to dogs, whose natural body weight generally varies between twenty and fifty kilos as an adult (Bouw 1991). The extent of this genetic manipulation and breeders' bid to achieve and surpass breed standards has often resulted in significant problems for animal well-being. Today, for example, the heads of bulldogs have become so large that bitches can have considerable difficulty giving birth and puppies must be delivered by caesarean section. Likewise, the majestic looking Great Dane has been bred to be so large that its heart cannot cope and usually gives up the ghost by the time the animal reaches the age of seven. Such problems are, however, not entirely a product of the intensification of breeding practices during the twentieth century. The deliberate selection of such traits became problematic during the late nineteenth century as dogs were crippled in breeders' vain attempts to meet breed standards (Ritvo 1987b: 163).

Cats, on the other hand, have largely escaped the wholesale genetic manipulation to which dogs have been subjected; at least, that is, until very recently. For many centuries, cats have lived alongside us, although their relationship with human beings has often been rather tenuous. In the course of human and feline history, cats have at times been venerated, but more often than not they have been barely tolerated or reviled, becoming the unfortunate victims of human distrust, superstition and barbarous entertainment. The dawn of the Enlightenment heralded a new era of tolerance for the cat as belief in necromancy declined and sensibilities towards animals gradually grew, but it was only during the late nineteenth century that cat fancy was actually established in western Europe and cats began, on a grand scale, to be transformed from scrawny feral street creatures into the fat lap-cats that today commonly lurk in our homes and gardens. The comparatively late acceptance of the cat as a suitable human companion has contributed to the fact that the modern domestic cat differs remarkably little from its wild conspecifics and ancestors. Modern breeders seem, however, to be making up for lost time and, in recent years, designer-made cats – bred on the basis of physical mutations – without coats, with squashed noses, curled back ears and even shortened legs have appeared (Clutton-Brock 1988; Tabor 1991).

Breeding has in fact always been an important facet of

pet-keeping, particularly where dogs are concerned. Since ancient times, a hierarchy amongst hounds has existed; dog breeds, it seems, mirroring social breeding. Historically speaking, the greyhound has generally been ranked number one in the canine charts. During the mediaeval period, no-one under the social rank of gentleman or free-holder was even permitted to own such a beast (Youatt 1845). Other hunting and fowling dogs, such as spaniels, have usually occupied the second rank position within this canine hierarchy, while lap-dogs – too small to be of any value for hunting purposes, but favoured by noblewomen and bourgeois ladies – have taken third place. Less attractive, though nonetheless useful, breeds, such as mastiffs and sheepdogs, have been regarded as being of yet lower status. And, finally, the currish cross-breeds kept by common folk have always found themselves at the bottom of the pile, being regarded as ugly creatures of no real use to humankind (e.g. Caius 1576; Ash 1927). Dogs were thus generally ranked according to their importance to the elite. The breeds with the greatest hunting prowess and aesthetic beauty were placed far above the working and mongrel dogs kept by people of lower social standing.

During the nineteenth century, this social division of dogs became embedded in the social rhetoric of the time, particularly as contemporary commentators began to paint an increasingly vivid image of the moral qualities and character of the canine species. As Ritvo – writing on Victorian England – observes, even the legal conventions of this age bestowed a hierarchy of moral attributes on dogs, associating both the calibre and character of animals with their owners (Ritvo 1987). A similar situation could be observed in nineteenth-century France, suggesting that this attribution of morality to animals was found beyond the shores of the British Isles (Kete 1994). While pet animals had become a fixed and cherished feature of many a bourgeois home, the respectable classes looked on the practice of pet-keeping amongst the poor with considerable disdain. The pet dogs of the poor were viewed as a wanton luxury for people who could not afford to adequately feed and clothe their families. Moreover, the presence of dogs in the squalid and insalubrious domiciles and establishments of the poor further emphasised the bourgeois sentiment of repugnance for the lower classes. One commentator, for example, wrote:

> In an economical point of view the diminution of the numbers of useless dogs is most desirable, and from a sanitary point of view even more essential. Useless dogs are

> badly kept by poor people, and are allowed to run about dirty and diseased. They are a source of waste and insalubrity, as they absorb the already insufficient supply of oxygen in the miserable and badly-ventilated dwellings of their owners, and they consume a certain quantity of food that can ill be spared.
>
> (Dolan 1879: 201–2)

According to the bourgeois view, poor people should be discouraged from keeping such animals by the imposition of taxes on such useless dogs and introduction of dog licences. As Ritvo has suggested, the bourgeoisie had found a new way for controlling at least one aspect of the urban human and canine proletariat (Ritvo 1987a: 186–9). However, it was not only the dogs of the poor that caught the attention of the Victorian middle class. It has been argued that the excesses of the rich were equally epitomised by the dogs that they kept. The aristocracy did not adhere to the same degree of moderation and restraint in their conduct as the affluent middle classes, and were thus singled out for their unruliness and lack of productivity. Such views were strongly reflected in contemporary views about rabies to which the dogs of both the poor and the rich were believed to be most susceptible (Ritvo 1987a; Swabe 1995). For example, the pampering and overfeeding of 'useless', 'inbred' small dogs by their aristocratic mistresses was thought to give them a predisposition to the disease (Dolan 1879: 202). Into the twentieth century, this kind of social rhetoric appears to have gradually diminished, most likely due to the increasing differentiation within society, which has led to the contrasts between individuals becoming less evident. The association of both social class and gender with particular dog breeds has, however, to some extent persisted; partially, I am inclined to argue, through stereotyping. Toy dogs continue to be associated with wealthy middle-aged women, whereas more 'macho' breeds such as bull terriers are associated with working-class males. While some kind of correlation between breed ownership and animal owners may indeed be possible, it is perhaps more appropriate to suggest that animals may be specifically kept to make a statement about the owner and his personality; a pet can, in fact, function as a status symbol.

Throughout the twentieth century, the popularity of pet animals has continued to grow, accelerating beyond all proportions since the end of the Second World War. The increasing material affluence of the post-war period has undoubtedly played a significant role in the growth of the pet population. In today's industrial society, keeping animals of no utilitarian value is seldom frowned on as a luxury. Individuals from all social strata can now afford to keep small animals for the companionship or whatever else they might offer. Moreover, there is a whole industry that exists today to service the needs and desires of pet owners both rich and poor. Pet-keeping as a practice is nowadays more or less taken for granted, though it is true to say that not everybody shares the passion or inclination that many people have for keeping animals in the home. Just as in centuries past, the affectionate bonds that can exist between pet and owner may today be criticised or ridiculed by others who fail to appreciate the joys of pet-keeping. One of the greatest criticisms of pet owners relates to the, sometimes disproportionate, amount of money that they are prepared to spend on their pets. Amongst the main beneficiaries of pet owners' pennies are the veterinary professionals who look after their animals' health. In the following, I shall examine the extension of the veterinary regime to pet animals, tracing the development of small-animal medicine from antiquity to the present day and exploring the role of the small-animal practitioner in protecting pet animal health and welfare.

Extending the veterinary regime to small animals

Today, the veterinarian clad in a pristine white coat expertly examining a pet pussy-cat or pooch on a surgical table is a familiar image, even to those who have never owned a pet or visited a veterinary surgery. Yet the role of the veterinarian as the defender of canine and feline health is a very recent one. Historically speaking, the diseases and afflictions of dogs and cats have received very limited veterinary attention. Unlike horses and livestock, whose inherent economic and nutritional value has motivated human attempts to preserve their health and cure their disease, these small domesticates and their attendant diseases have posed little threat to the human economy or public health; this is, of course, with the exception of one highly notorious zoonotic disease: *rabies* – which will be discussed shortly.

In centuries past, dogs and cats simply did not warrant the therapeutic attentions of medical science; while useful creatures – for protection, pest control and companionship – they were essentially of little economic value and were easily replaceable. Instead, the architects of medical science saw the canine species in a quite different light as the ideal subjects for the experimental study of anatomy and physiology; dogs were, after all, cheap, abundant and easy for the experimenters to control. Further to this, small animals – or rather parts or by-products of them – provided the useful ingredients for the medical pharmacopoeia of the past (Boor-van der Putten 1986: 9–10). The thirteenth-century encyclopaedist Albertus Magnus, for example, reports that 'dried dog dung, taken orally, has a constricting effect on the bowels, especially when the dung has been collected from dogs which gnaw on bones and it has been dried in the sun for twenty days during the month of July'. To achieve the best results, he advises that one should 'take one quarter of an ounce of dried dog faeces, mix it with the broth obtained by boiling an old rooster, and consume this liquid before sunrise'. This same medication was also claimed to be effective in treating laryngitis and tonsillar abscesses. Likewise, he recounts the interesting claim that 'urinary incontinence can be prevented by carrying the skin of a dog's penis which has been wrapped around some soil on which a human has urinated' (Albertus Magnus 1987: 86–7).

Yet while medical science had a tendency to use small animals either as the objects of anatomical study or as the provider of potentially useful ingredients to cure human ailments, there is evidence that they did sometimes receive a degree of therapeutic attention and care, generally in accordance with their usefulness. In the agriculturally based society of ancient Rome, for example, shepherd and guard dogs played an important role in protecting both humans and their livestock and property. Columella, for example, sings the praises of the dog by advising his readers 'in a word, who will be more steady in avenging your injuries, or protecting you from them? Wherefore a Husbandman ought to purchase and maintain this animal, even among the very first things, because he keeps and guards both the manor-house, and the fruits, and the family and the cattle' (Columella 1745: 332). In this spirit, he offered a number of remedies for the prevention of ticks and fleas and cures for the ulceration and scab that may accompany infestations. For example, he suggested that a dog plagued by fleas can be treated with 'either cumin bruised in an equal quantity with white hellebore, and mixed with water, and rubbed on them; or the juice of a serpentine cucumber' (Columella 1745: 336–7). It is possible that such folk remedies were commonly employed in the care and management of working dogs during ancient times, though there is little evidence of how widespread such treatments were or how seriously canine health was actually taken.

Perhaps the most fertile source of historical information on the early care and diseases of dogs can be found in the mediaeval literature on hunting and hawking. During the middle ages, the art of hunting and falconry enjoyed great popularity amongst the nobility of feudal Europe. The care of hunting hounds and birds became increasingly important and demanded the attentions of specialist animal attendants who could oversee the health and care of these valued creatures (Boor-van der Putten 1986: 13). Kennel boys in fact began learning their trade from the age of seven and were fully accomplished in all aspects of canine care and preparation for hunting parties by the time they reached fourteen (Boor-van der Putten 1990: 61). The specialist knowledge they acquired and practised was eventually recorded in a number of works devoted to hunting which appeared from the fourteenth century onwards; the most celebrated of those was the *Livre de Chasse*, penned by Gaston Phebus, Count of Foix-Béarn. This exquisitely illustrated book was translated into English by the Duke of York, appearing under the title *The Master of the Game* (ca. 1406–13); and was further reworked during the mid-sixteenth century by du Fouilloux as *La Vénerie*, which in turn was translated, or rather plagiarised, by Turberville as *The Noble art of Venerie or Hunting* (1575). Phebus' book, therefore, formed the basis for knowledge of hunting and the care of hunting hounds for centuries to come (Boor-van der Putten 1990: 60–1).

The *Livre de Chasse* is particularly revealing, not only for the beautiful illustrations that depict both hunting scenes and the care and treatment of dogs, but also for the detail it offers on canine nutrition, disease and therapy. In contrast to earlier texts, Phebus went further than simply providing a list of recipes for curing canine conditions. For example, he described the necessity of isolating dogs suffering from scabies and also the surgical removal of the third eyelid, a membrane that can grow over an animal's eye leading eventually to blindness. Furthermore, he detailed the treatment of wounds and fractures, in addition to the castration of animals which, he advises, should be performed by a professional castrator (Boor-van der Putten 1990: 63–5). Phebus' work gives an impression of the kind of care and attention that the (privileged) hunting hounds of the nobility might have received during their lifetimes. However, it remains unclear what kind of therapeutic care the less well-bred dogs of the peasantry would have received. Indeed, it is said that the dogs of ordinary folk, who lived in the vicinity of the royal forests where the nobility would hunt game, were forcibly mutilated in order that they could not assist their owners in any poaching they might attempt (Dunlop and Williams 1996: 229).

Mad dogs and medicine

Common to all early texts that deal – however briefly – with the canine condition is an overwhelming concern for rabies and its prevention. Unlike other canine afflictions, rabies is a disease, which although uncommon, has always posed a direct threat – albeit often imagined – to the health of both humans and their livestock. From antiquity onwards, the image of the mad dog and the ravages of the disease on its human victims have deeply affected the human condition, inspiring not only great fear and trepidation, but also prejudice and irrationality; much of which has been embodied by the folklore that has surrounded the disease since ancient times. Rabies is in fact one of the oldest infectious diseases known to humankind and has occupied a unique, yet curious, place within disease history. From the earliest accounts of rabies, writers established a clear causal link between the disease and the saliva accompanying a dog bite. Although it was recognised from early times that other species could be affected by the disease, rabies has always been associated with dogs. This is perhaps not without good reason; as the German naturalist Paullinus remarked in 1677, the disease was commonly known as '*Rabies Canina* not because it is inflicted by dogs alone, or because dogs are only seized by this disease . . . but because dogs are much more subject to it and to a greater degree than all other animals, and because living along with us as domestic animals, they all the more easily communicate the evil to us' (Ash 1927: 654).

The speculation and folklore that has surrounded rabies since ancient times was frequently translated into practice by those seeking to protect their hounds – and consequently themselves – from the ravages of rabies. For example, during the Roman era, shepherds commonly believed that docking their dogs' tails would prevent the animals from developing the 'madness' (Columella 1745).[1] Another anti-rabies practice, also apparently deriving from Roman times, was the removal of the *frenum linguae*, the mucous membrane that attaches the dog's tongue. It was commonly believed that this membrane was a worm that should be removed when the animal was a pup to prevent it becoming mad in later life. The natural scientist, Pliny the Elder, had already advised that this 'worm' be given to those who had been bitten by mad dogs in order to preserve their sanity. The notion of the tongue-worm persisted well into the nineteenth century, much to the chagrin of later and more enlightened veterinary experts. For example, writing in the 1880s, Benjamin Clayton scorned this 'very old and strange prejudice', arguing that 'the notion is perfectly absurd, and many dogs are put to unnecessary torture, as the extraction of the harmless ligament, which has been elevated to the dignity of a worm, is an extremely painful operation' (Clayton 188?: 26).

Throughout history, therefore, dogs have been subjected to a wide variety of indignities in the bid to deal with the disease. Perhaps the most barbaric, however, is recorded in Albertus Magnus' *De Animalibus*. Here the author recounts that

> according to the writings of Ameria, King of Valentia, a rabid dog should be immersed in a tank of hot water, suspended by its forepaws so that the hind feet barely touch the bottom; and the entire length of its body should be submerged for nine days. After removal from the water, its head and body should be shaved, even to the extent of scarifying the skin. Then, it should be smeared with beet juice and re-dipped in the tank for additional immersion. If the dog eats at all during this period, its food should be marinated in beet juice and mixed with the pitch of black elder, because the latter is also beneficial. However, if no favourable results are obtained in the next seven days, the dog should be slain, for it will never be cured.
>
> (Albertus Magnus 1987: 84–5)

Speculation about the causes of rabies and its possible cure persisted long after the Middle Ages. The first publication believed to be specifically devoted to the topic of rabies appeared in 1613. Penned by an English physician, Thomas Spackman, *A declaration of such grievous accidents as commonly follow the biting of mad dogges*, promoted the popular idea of the spontaneous generation of rabies in dogs, noting that the 'inward causes' of canine rabies were an excess of heat and cold, insufficient water and a 'peculiar natural propensity' of dogs to go mad. Adding a number of 'external causes', he noted that contagion could occur through being bitten, from feeding on carrion or animals that have died from plague or rot, or have been killed by lightning. To this list, he even included the grief that a dog might suffer at the loss of his master as a cause. Spackman also suggested that black and red coloured dogs were more prone to the disease, as were likewise hair-coloured men and women (Spackman 1613: 12–22).

Theories on and cures for rabies continued to abound into the eighteenth and nineteenth centuries. During this period, numerous essays and treatises on the subject were published, particularly with reference to its transmission to humans (e.g. James 1760; Layard 1762; Murray 1830; Shadwell 1790; White 1862; Wood 1814; Youatt 1830). It was at this time that human fears of contracting rabies from their canine companions appeared to reach a greater virulence than the virus itself. As consequence, dogs – particularly those of the lower classes – were subject to fanatical persecution during the nineteenth century and hundreds of them were martyred under even the slightest hint of them suffering from madness. It is in fact likely that the majority of these unfortunate mutts suffered from fits or encephalitis, a symptom of canine distemper, rather than rabies; alternatively, they were simply condemned because they were just plain 'unpleasant looking' (Ritvo 1987a; Swabe 1995). This confusion of the symptoms of rabies with those of other canine conditions, as frequently occurred during the nineteenth century, begs the question of whether many of the mad animals that have been described in the literature dating back to antiquity were actually suffering from rabies at all.

Whatever the case, it was only towards the close of the nineteenth century that human fears about the threat of canine rabies appear to have been attenuated. During the 1880s, Pasteur's experiments at last conclusively proved that rabies could only be transmitted by inoculation, ultimately dealing a death blow to the previously popular theories on spontaneous generation. The prognosis for humans bitten by a rabid animal was also radically improved by Pasteur's development of a post-exposure vaccine. Since that time, public health measures and legislation designed to eradicate the rabies virus, in addition to quarantine measures, border controls and the widespread vaccination of pet populations, have greatly reduced the threat of rabies to both human and pet populations within Europe.

Nineteenth-century innovations in small-animal medicine

While rabies seems to have preoccupied the hearts and minds of many a writer throughout the ages, other aspects of canine care and disease seem to have generally been overlooked. Certainly, from the sixteenth century onwards, there were a number of publications devoted exclusively to the dog – e.g. Caius' *Of Englishe Dogges* (1576) and Paullinus' *Cynographia Curiosa* (1677 – referred to in Ash 1927) – but these were more greatly concerned with describing the wide variety of breeds and their functions, rather than specifically addressing issues of canine health. It was only in 1783 that the first popular work specifically devoted to the diseases of the dog appeared, written by the empiricist John Clater (Boor-van der Putten 1986: 15). During the early nineteenth century, additional works dedicated exclusively to the veterinary treatment and understanding of canine disease were published. However, as Delabere Blaine – the self-styled patriarch of canine medicine – remarked in the preface to his pioneering work *Canine Pathology* (1817), devoting time and energy to this subject inevitably met with considerable social disapprobation. He lamented that 'my attention to the medical treatment of dogs subjected me to an imputation of want of common pride, and an utter disrespect for my former character and habits'. Certainly – as illustrated in Chapter 4 – the prevailing view at that time was that animal medicine was not only greatly inferior to human medicine, but also that the horse was the *only* species of animal that was believed to deserve *any* veterinary medical attention whatsoever.

Yet while the fledgling veterinary profession in general failed to acknowledge the importance of employing its skills and directing its attention to the diseases of dogs and other small animals, with the rise in the practice of pet-keeping there was evidently a growing market for professional advice on this very subject. Blaine clearly recognised this and found himself a niche in the market as an animal doctor, author on canine health and purveyor of veterinary medicines. Interestingly, he was never actually a qualified veterinarian, although as a former surgeon's apprentice and anatomical artist, he had worked briefly as an assistant to Charles Vial de St Bel – the founder of the London Veterinary College. Blaine acquired much of his veterinary experience as a surgeon in the horse artillery, where he tended both human and equine patients. As a consequence of his experience treating horses, he produced a work on equine anatomy in 1799. The following year, he published *A Concise Description of the Distemper in Dogs, With an Account of the Discovery of an Efficacious Remedy for It* (1800). Essentially, this book was a blatant attempt to promote his own remedy for canine distemper, recognised today as a serious viral disease – related to measles in humans and rinderpest in cattle – which results in great mortality amongst puppies and young dogs. However, it does provide considerable clinical detail on the disease and Blaine clearly points out that the symptoms that accompany this disease can frequently be mistaken for 'madness' (Blaine 1800: 18).

The popularity and success of this publication inspired him to set up a veterinary practice in London and he continued to write extensively on both the diseases and anatomy of both horses and dogs, in addition to patenting various other medicinal purging balls and powders for curing canine distemper, mange, worms, etc. Blaine was, however, shunned by the veterinary establishment as a quack, though he is today regarded by veterinary historians as a visionary for his detailed attention to canine disease (Dunlop and Williams 1996: 597). Blaine was also exceptional in that he rejected the principles of humoral pathology that were prevalent amongst his contemporaries, in favour of the study of pathological anatomy. Clearly this rational medical approach was later more widely valued as *Canine Pathology* eventually underwent several reprints throughout the nineteenth century and was translated into French, German and Italian (Boor-van der Putten 1986: 21–2). Interestingly, Blaine also appears to have been one of the first authors to address the issue of feline disease. At the end of *Canine Pathology*, he wrote that though cats

> are very inferior, in all their properties, to dogs, yet they are not only useful to mankind, but as being domesticated with him, humanity is very materially concerned in a due attention to their welfare and comfort. Cats are subject to but a few diseases compared with the number entailed on dogs; one principal reason for which appears to be, that domestication had done little towards reclaiming their natural habits: and hence they are less subjected to the variations in health that are consequent to a life of art. But a still more cogent reason may possibly be found in the inferiority of their natures in the scale of animated existence.
>
> (Blaine 1817: 175)

Although regarding these creatures as inferior, he described various conditions from which cats may suffer; for example, fits, worms and distemper (feline panleukopenia) – which, he adds, ravaged across Europe in 1803, killing an estimated half of the cat population. Blaine describes the procedure of castrating a cat, which indeed is in many respects similar to the present-day operation. To perform this operation, he suggests that the cat be secured by either being put with its head and fore-quarters into a boot, or by rolling the body lengthways in several yards of towelling.

By 1813, Blaine had acquired a partner in crime: William Youatt. Like Blaine, Youatt was passionate about dogs, though he had neither veterinary nor medical experience when he joined Blaine's practice as an apprentice at the age of thirty-seven. He was encouraged by his mentor to join the Royal Veterinary College, in order to obtain a legitimate diploma, but was eventually hounded out by the then principal, Professor Coleman; a man with whom Blaine had persistently been in conflict for reducing veterinary training to but a few months, instead of the three years that St Bel had originally intended. Youatt wrote prolifically throughout his career, not only on the subject of canine medicine, but also on a variety of domesticated species; later becoming the editor of *The Veterinarian*, a journal that was most influential to the development of veterinary medicine in Britain (Wilkinson 1992: 98). After Coleman's death, and just three years before his own, Youatt was finally awarded his veterinary diploma by the Royal College of Veterinary Surgeons.

Youatt's best-known publication, *The Dog* (1845), provides an interesting history of dog-keeping and offers detailed descriptions of breeds, though it was clearly written with notions of biblical creation and ideas of the servitude of animals in mind. In this vein, he declares that the dog 'was the one animal whose service [to man] was voluntary, and who was susceptible of disinterested affection and gratitude' (Youatt 1845: 1). Within this volume, Youatt goes into considerable detail on the conditions and diseases of the dog and their treatment. In his chapter on rabies, he scornfully rejects the theories of spontaneous generation still espoused, amongst others, by the leading veterinary figures within Europe, emphasising clearly that it can only be caused by inoculation alone. This resonates the opinions expressed in an earlier publication *On Canine Madness* (1830), a tract within which Youatt does not shy away from expressing a moral opinion, linking the propagation of rabies to 'the increasing demoralisation of the country', specifically in relation to such nefarious activities as poaching and dog-fighting. In this respect, he called for the introduction of a tax to be levied on all 'useless' dogs, with extra penalties for owners if they were found loose or used for fighting (Youatt 1830: 30). Youatt's stature as a humanitarian and defender of kindness to animals, however, shines through in his work. He is, for example, highly critical of the indignities through which nineteenth-century dogs were put to suit the whims of their owners. With regard to tail-docking, he writes:

> [t]hen the tail of the dog does not suit the fancy of the owner. It must be shortened in some of these animals, and taken off altogether in others. If the sharp, strong scissors, with a ligature, were used, the operation, although still indefensible, would not be a very cruel one, for the tail may be removed in almost a moment, and the wound soon heals; but for the beastly gnawing off of the part – and drawing out the tendons and nerves – these are the acts of a cannibal; and he who orders or perpetrates a barbarity so nearly approaching to cannibalism deserves to be scouted from all society.
>
> (Youatt 1845: 112)

Blaine and Youatt's successful London practice provided the incentive for other veterinary surgeons to follow suit and open up specialist veterinary practices for dogs in other cities. Yet while the market for canine veterinary services gradually expanded within Britain, the question remained of whether the diploma-wielding veterinarians of the London Veterinary College and its Edinburgh counterpart (that had been established in 1823) truly possessed the competence and skills necessary to treat dogs. For, in spite of the duo's innovations and the increasing popularity of pet-keeping, veterinary education continued to remain firmly focused on the treatment of horses and – to a much lesser extent – livestock species. In the majority of nineteenth-century textbooks that were produced to assist veterinary training, the dog and its complaints generally only received a cursory mention. It was only in 1888 that the first book dedicated to canine disease and designed explicitly for veterinary teaching purposes was published by J.H. Steel. By the mid to late nineteenth century, the market for specialist canine veterinary services emerged within mainland Europe and North America. In cities such as Amsterdam and The Hague, for instance, urban veterinary practices were established to deal exclusively with dogs and horses (Boor-van der Putten 1986: 17–25). Small-animal medicine was, however, still very much in its infancy; it was only during the course of the twentieth century that it would come of age.

The twentieth-century expansion of small-animal practice

At the turn of the century, the attitude of the veterinary profession was still largely ambivalent towards the whole idea of studying and treating pet animals and their diseases. The increasing sentimentality towards animals, particularly amongst the urban middle classes, seems to have been quite alien to most veterinary practitioners who only saw profit, both in monetary and societal terms, in treating creatures of clear economic value. This attitude was also echoed throughout the veterinary schools of Europe, which continued to regard the study and treatment of small animals with considerable disdain. The veterinary profession had after all striven hard throughout the nineteenth century to elevate itself far above the 'vulgar' level of gelders and blacksmiths and wished to be taken seriously as a scientifically enlightened and socially useful profession (Porter 1993: 28–9); these educated veterinarians did not now wish to lower themselves by tending to, what they essentially regarded as, 'useless' animals (Offringa 1983).

One of the chief consequences of this attitude was that, at least until the dawn of the twentieth century, there was comparatively little knowledge of or concern for the nature and pathology of small-animal disease. Up until this time, veterinary attention to this subject seems to have only been justified when the study of small-animal disease was seen as instrumental to increasing understanding of the pathology of horses or food-producing animals (Boor-van der Putten 1986: 236). More significantly still, most of the advancement that occurred in understanding the diseases and physiology of small animals occurred indirectly through scientific research aimed at understanding and improving human health. For example, experiments conducted on dogs led to the understanding of the process of endocrine secretion in humans, eventually resulting in the isolation of insulin during the 1920s. It was, however, to take many years before such discoveries were actually applied in the treatment of dogs and cats (Dunlop and Williams 1996: 600–1).

Yet while pet animals were regarded with a great deal of contempt by the veterinary establishment, they nonetheless seem to have insidiously crept into the veterinary schools as patients. From the late nineteenth century onwards, increasing numbers of small animals and birds were brought by their owners to the veterinary schools for treatment at out-patients' clinics, eventually necessitating the establishment of accommodation for animals requiring hospitalisation. In the Netherlands, for example, the Rijksveeartsenijschool (State Veterinary School) in Utrecht witnessed a steady increase in the numbers of dogs, cats and birds that could not be ignored. By 1881, dogs made up the greatest part of the patient body on which the School's vets could practise their clinical skills. In quantitative terms, therefore, dogs had become the most important group of animal patients visiting the school. The clinicians, however, continued to look down on these patients, still preferring to treat the larger and, to them, inherently more interesting patients such as horses and cattle, that attended the same out-patients' clinics in lesser numbers. Perhaps as a measure of the lack of native interest in small-animal medicine, when the Rijksveeartsenijschool eventually took steps to establish a special clinic for small animals, they had to look to Germany to find a veterinary practitioner capable of heading it. Heinrich Jakob's appointment to the school in 1911 heralded a new era for veterinary education within the Netherlands, with a new emphasis on clinical examination and a higher regard for the diseases and pathology of small animals (Boor-van der Putten 1986: 51–65).

Elsewhere in Europe, the veterinary interest in small animals also continued to grow along with the numbers of canine, feline and avian patients demanding veterinary attention. Britain, in particular, continued to produce innovators in this area and new technologies emerged that would later become essential to small-animal practice. For instance, the development of anaesthesia during the mid-nineteenth century provided veterinary medicine with a new tool to assist surgery. The first experiments with ether anaesthesia on dogs and cats were performed by Edward Mayhew (Dunlop and Williams 1996: 606). Later, Frederick Hobday – who, at the turn of the century, was in charge of the free out-patients' clinic at the Royal Veterinary College, London – succeeded in developing a method whereby anaesthetic vapours could be administered to dogs in a far safer manner than ever before. His publication *Canine and Feline Surgery* (1900) outlines how the various surgical techniques, administration of anaesthesia, securing of patients, etc., of that era were performed. In this text, there is fine attention paid to the necessity of hygiene, both personal and of surgical instruments, and the use of antiseptics to avoid bacterial infection. Hobday was also responsible for introducing Roentgen's X-ray technology to the London veterinary school as an aid to veterinary diagnosis. By 1927, he had been appointed as principal of the Royal

Veterinary College, signalling a new era of openness towards small-animal medicine in British veterinary education.

However, in spite of both the increasing numbers of pet animals requiring treatment and the emerging medical technologies and innovators able to provide it, the rise of small-animal medicine during the twentieth century perhaps owes greater thanks to the invention of the internal combustion engine than anything else. The rise of motorised transport – as discussed in the previous chapter – led to the inevitable decline of the importance of the horse in European society. This development had its greatest consequences for the urban veterinary practitioners who had, until then, made their living by tending the horses of private citizens, local businesses and the local municipality. But as the horses that pulled the carriages, wagons, carts, trams and even the fire-brigade were replaced by motorised vehicles, the urban veterinarians were left with little local work other than meat inspection (Offringa 1981: 41). Thus it was more by accident than design that the veterinary practitioners of the early twentieth century set aside their contempt for small animals and instead began to earn a living from them.

After the First World War, increasingly more practices devoted exclusively to the veterinary treatment of small animals were established in urban areas, generally deriving their income and clientele from the more affluent middle-class denizens of the community. Special small-animal clinics were sometimes established in league with animal protection organisations and the newly emerging animal sanctuaries to provide veterinary care for pet animals (Davids 1989: 92). This trend continued with a vengeance after the end of the Second World War. As the above discussion has already shown, the practice of pet-keeping rapidly increased in popularity during the post-war period. The increased material affluence of post-war society has not only influenced our tendency to keep pets, but has also provided us with the means to go to considerable lengths to ensure their lives are happy and healthy ones. During the past fifty years or so, an entire industry has sprung up to provide and service pet animal needs. From the breeders who produce tailor-made animals to the pet food manufacturers who feed them, it has been realised that there are considerable profits to be made by exploiting our attachment to small animals and encouraging people to keep them as pets. The veterinary world has not been immune to this development and consequently small-animal medicine has rapidly become the most progressive area within veterinary medicine; it has also become a rather profitable one. This is indeed a far cry from a mere century ago when dogs and cats were more or less shunned by the veterinary profession.

In this respect, perhaps one of the most interesting developments in veterinary medical science during the twentieth century has been the rise of feline medicine. As has already been illustrated, until the late nineteenth century, small animal medicine was essentially entirely equatable with canine medicine: cats did not get much of a look in. During the early twentieth century, veterinary researchers chose only really to focus on feline diseases that were hazardous to human health, e.g. toxoplasmosis, tuberculosis, rather than the feline condition *per se*. Since the late 1920s, increasing scientific attention has been paid to panleukopenia and the other viral infections that afflict cats, leading to the development and widespread application of effective vaccines. More recently, specific attention has been paid to both nutrition and behavioural problems in cats (Dunlop and Williams 1996: 615–17). Given that cats have today surpassed dogs in the popularity stakes, it is likely that in the future feline health will receive increasing veterinary attention. The rise of feline medicine also reflects the degree of specialisation with which veterinary medicine during the twentieth century can be characterised.

It is also important to note that during the post-war period, the small-animal practitioner has not merely been confined to urban practice, but can be routinely found in rural practices. Although veterinary education has become increasingly specialised throughout the past decades, all veterinarians are qualified to treat both agricultural and pet animals. During the later stages of their training, prospective vets can decide the course of their future vocation and elect to specialise in large- or small-animal practice. Although many rural practices may employ a small-animal specialist, the livestock or equine specialist may indeed also be responsible for treating the pet animals of the local population; a substantial proportion of which, although resident in a rural area, are today not directly involved in agriculture and share similar sentiments about their pets to their urban counterparts. By the same token, the urban veterinarian may at times also be required to treat large animals in city farms and stables. The daily life of a veterinarian can therefore be extremely varied. The animal doctor who delivers a beef-bred calf by caesarean section in a cow shed in the early hours of the morning may well, only hours later, scrub up and don a pristine white coat to examine and treat the pampered pets of the local community.

In this respect, the great disparity in treatment, both cultural and medical, of domesticated animals can be observed within daily veterinary practice; at least within the small mixed rural practice. Although, as will shortly be discussed, the small-animal practitioner is similarly overwhelmingly concerned with preventative medical treatment and the management of animal (re)production as was the large animal practitioner discussed in the previous chapter, there appears to be far more room for manoeuvre within small-animal medicine with regard to therapy and cure, than in large-animal medicine; and, more importantly, unlike livestock, small animals are treated very much as individuals. In recent years, the extent of people's emotional attachment to pet animals means that they are frequently prepared to spend vast amounts of money to keep their cherished animals alive and well for as long as possible. This can sometimes go to great extremes when an animal's quality of life is significantly reduced and an owner refuses to consider euthanasia as a viable option, even though it is both in his or her interests financially and in the animal's interests with regard to its enjoyment of life and physical condition (cf. Swabe 1994, 1996).

This is, of course, in stark contrast to the lot of food-producing animals who will only receive veterinary treatment, particularly operative, on the basis of their economic value, age and future potential economic capacity, in addition to the nature of the sickness or injury. Today, there is such a demand and market for small-animal veterinary services that the profession has been able to specialise in a fashion akin to human medicine, thus providing a range of therapeutic options unavailable – or rather uneconomical – to the treatment of large animals. Thus, if one's cat has cancer, it may not simply only be operated on to remove the offending tumour, but it might also receive chemotherapy. Likewise, it is today commonplace for clients to bring rabbits, guinea-pigs and other rodents, not to mention reptiles, for veterinary treatment; in the not too distant past this would also have been unthinkable. Nowadays, there are a growing number of veterinary specialists who operate outside the realms of the veterinary schools where the employment of innovative techniques and medical specialisation are commonplace. One can today, for example, consult veterinary specialists in internal medicine, dermatology, radiography, dentistry, orthopaedics, homeopathy, acupuncture, etc. The market for such services is there and some, but by no means all, pet-owners are prepared to pay for them. It is largely for this reason that small-animal practitioners make up the largest group within the veterinary profession today, women making up an increasing proportion of the group.

A mere century ago, taking one's dog or cat to the veterinarian was more the exception than the rule; today, it is a completely normal state of affairs. In recent decades, the importance of preserving pet health seems to have become deeply embedded in our habitus. To this we can perhaps partially owe the plethora of literature, films, documentaries and television series that have been produced highlighting and endearing the role of the veterinarian to wider society. The popular image of the kindly animal doctor has become firmly fixed in our collective imagination and has been repeatedly reinforced by the images that are routinely broadcast into our living rooms. The TV vet, be he real or fictional, is a sight now familiar to all; moreover, he brings with him particular public expectations of the profession (Singleton 1993: 255). Their example has perhaps reinforced our inclination to pay attention to our pets' behaviour and health, and thus more readily seek veterinary help if they exhibit unusual or worrying symptoms of disease. It can be argued that the media preoccupation with animals and animal medicine has also to some extent facilitated the process of proto-professionalisation of veterinary medicine amongst lay people (de Swaan 1988: 144–6).

Essentially, proto-professionalisation means that animal owners have become increasingly familiar with the basic notions and practices of the veterinary profession. They will borrow professional veterinary vocabulary to articulate their animal's health or behavioural problems and will use their knowledge of animal conditions to determine whether or not they should solicit veterinary assistance. With this increased lay knowledge, animal owners may tend to view veterinary professionals more critically, which in turn places increased pressure on veterinarians to demonstrate their competence and medical expertise to their clients and to retain their medical authority. The proto-professionalisation of animal owners, combined with the more general public fascination with animals and veterinary work, has, however, greatly helped the veterinary profession to reinforce and transmit the necessity of vaccinating the pet population against serious infectious diseases, such as parvovirus, canine distemper, infectious canine hepatitis, feline panleukopenia, viral rhinotracheitis, leptospirosis and rabies, and treating animals for worms and other parasitic infestations. For many pet-owners, it has now become routine to pay an annual visit to the vet's to have their animals vaccinated, along with a general check-up. Consultations for vaccination and parasite control in fact account for a great proportion of the small-animal practitioner's daily activities and income. Animal disease control is, therefore, as large a part of the routine work of the small-animal practitioner as of the rural veterinarian.

The pet industry has greatly contributed to the promotion of small-animal health in recent decades. From the production of specialist pet foods for overweight pets to anti-flea products, to even pet health insurance schemes and the specially designed plastic boxes in which one's pet can be transported to the veterinary surgery, they have created increasingly more ways for pet-owners to part with their pennies in order to take care of their animals. The pet industry, however, bears some of the responsibility for some of the most serious problems to face pet animal species, certainly as far as breeders and many pet shops are concerned. Animals, wholly unsuited to their new owners or the living environments they are able to offer them, are frequently sold and then discarded when either their owners realise they cannot cope with them, or when their novelty has worn off. During the past few decades, the pet population has grown enormously, the chief consequence of this being that as animal numbers continue to multiply, sanctuaries overflow with unwanted animals; some of which may be re-housed, others eventually euthanised. The skills of the veterinarian are in ever-increasing need in the bid to control the growth of pet animal populations through neutering. In recent years, there have been great attempts by both the veterinary establishment and animal welfare groups to educate the public with regard to the necessity of having their pets sterilised or castrated as young as possible. The responsibilities of pet-ownership are thus ever-increasingly being drummed into the public's mind and animal owners encouraged to participate actively within the veterinary regime.

Pets and human health: benefits and risks

As the above discussion clearly shows, the extension of the veterinary regime to small animals has become all the more important as our interactions and intimacy with them have increased. In the following, I shall focus more specifically on the relationship between pet-keeping and human health, since this is directly relevant to the intensification of the veterinary regime. Further to this, the impact of pet-keeping on the environment will be considered, given that this has considerable bearing on issues of public health.

In recent years, there has been increasing attention paid to the role which pet animals play in enhancing human well-being and quality of life (e.g. Anderson *et al*. 1984; Fogle 1981; Katcher and Beck 1983; Robinson 1995). Numerous studies have been conducted in order to gauge the beneficial effects that keeping or interacting with pets may have on both our physical and psychological health. Perhaps not so surprisingly, much of this academic research has been funded by the pet industry; in whose interest it has been to convince us that keeping small animals around our homes is good for us. Nonetheless, such research has been responsible for expanding our knowledge of how the interaction between humans and pet animals can affect both parties. There has, for example, been considerable attention paid to the positive psychological role that pet animals can play in child development (e.g. Levinson 1972; Endenburg and Baarda 1995). Likewise, the direct health benefits of interacting with small animals have become the focus of medical research. For instance, it has been found that pet-ownership can be a positive factor in the survival of patients suffering from coronary heart disease. In this respect, pets appear to be useful mediators of stress and can have a positive influence on people suffering from blood pressure, hypertension and heart disease (e.g. Friedmann *et al*. 1983; Friedmann 1995; Katcher 1981). Extensive research has also been conducted into the manner in which small animals can enhance the psychological and physical well-being of the elderly and other socially marginalised groups (e.g. Hart 1995). As a consequence, pet therapy and pet visiting schemes are today increasingly introduced to benefit people who are physically disabled or institutionalised in hospices, old people's homes and even prisons (CSS report 1988: 33–6). The results of such research into the psychological and physiological effects of pet ownership have filtered down from academia to the public level as the mass media have picked up on and widely publicised the health benefits of keeping animals as pets. However, although our associations with pet animals have, in some respects, clearly had a positive effect on our lives, there is a significant downside to this relationship with respect to environmental nuisance and infectious disease.

Like farm waste, pet animal excreta pose a particular problem for the environment and public health. The natural behaviour of dogs and the carelessness or thoughtlessness of dog owners in managing their canine charges have become an increasing bone of contention in many urban areas. Although local authorities across Europe have instituted a wide variety of measures to deal with this problem, people still fail to clear up after their animals or allow them to defecate freely. Apart from simply being unpleasant, the fouling of public places, particularly where children play, presents more serious problems. Coming into contact with pet animal faeces can potentially be quite hazardous for human health. In recent years, increasing attention has been paid to the dangers posed by the roundworm larvae that can be found in canine and, less frequently, feline excreta. Toxocariasis, a helminth infection, has perhaps been the most widely publicised disease transmitted through contact with pet animal faeces. *Toxocara canis* is also thought to be the most frequent zoonotic parasite that is acquired from dogs (Glickman 1993: 5). *Toxocara catus* poses a far lesser threat because the roundworm eggs that cats pass in their faeces only become infectious after about two weeks. Given that cats are particularly fastidious creatures, they tend not to leave excrement on their skin surfaces for long. Feline defecation in the sandboxes where children play presents the most significant opportunity for human infection to occur (Lappin 1993: 67). Toxocariasis is caused by migrating larvae and can result in blindness, disability or even death in humans; though severe cases of infection are rare (Bisseru 1967; Glickman 1993). In dogs and cats, the only clinical symptoms which they might display is some respiratory distress as the larvae migrate through their bodies; adult roundworms may cause loss of condition in the animal (Schwabe 1984a: 237). Contact with *T. canis* eggs in soil appears to play the most important role in the transmission of the disease to humans. Indeed, studies have even shown that fifty per cent of patients suffering from clinical toxocariasis had never even owned a dog or had close contacts with one (Lloyd 1993: 17). The enforcement of local laws to prevent environmental contamination with *T. canis* eggs, the education of animal owners to supervise and clean up after their dogs and the worming of puppies may greatly reduce the risk of human toxocariasis (Glickman 1993: 8–9).

Like toxocariasis, toxoplasmosis (a protozoal infection) – which, as has already been illustrated in previous chapters, is often associated with handling or eating raw meat – can be transmitted to humans and other mammals through contact with infected pet animal faeces. Although this infection can be picked up through contact with canine excrement, toxoplasmosis is more commonly associated with cat-keeping. Cats generally will acquire infection by ingesting uncooked meat from an intermediate host such as a rodent, or from the raw liver which is sometimes fed to cats to improve coat texture given that it is high in vitamin A. Because *Toxoplasma gondii* are often found in the livers of food-producing animals, cats should not be given such raw meat. Instead they should be fed only on dry, tinned or cooked foods (Dubey and Beattie 1988: 29). Cats usually display no clinical symptoms, so infection will not be apparent. They will, however, shed oocysts in their faeces – which can survive in the environment, particularly soil, for months or even years – and then be passed on to other animals through ingestion (Lappin 1993: 70). Failure to wash one's hands after emptying a cat's litter tray can, therefore, lead to infection, especially if food is prepared shortly afterwards. Likewise, it is advised that garden vegetables should be washed thoroughly before they are consumed, because they too may have been contaminated by cat faeces in the soil (Dubey and Beattie ibid.). As with many other infectious diseases, the adoption of a rigorous hygiene regime is the simplest way to prevent infection. *T. gondii* are most particularly hazardous to children and pregnant women, and deadly to people whose immune system has been compromised by conditions such as AIDS. Prenatal infection in humans can be fatal, while postnatal infection may result in encephalitis (Schwabe 1984a: 207). Cats infected with toxoplasmosis can pose potential problems in farm environments. Toxoplasmosis is sometimes the cause of abortion and neonatal mortality in sheep, so it is therefore advised that cats be kept away from pregnant ewes (Dubey and Beattie ibid.: 30).

The increasing popularity of keeping cats – particularly those confined to an indoor life – has created increasingly serious environmental problems during the past couple of decades. Deprived of natural surfaces on which they can defecate, cats must be provided with a tray in which they can do their business. Although one can simply use old newspaper in a litter tray, it is preferable for the cat to have gravel-like matter in which it can dig and cover up its excrement. Such cat litter is available not only at considerable expense to the cat owner, but also to the cost of the environment. For example, in the Netherlands, the immense popularity of the cat has meant that like farm waste, the country also has the biggest waste problem due to cat litter in the whole of Europe.[2] In 1995, the *Volkskrant* (27 June) reported that cats produce 100,000 tonnes of waste per annum; that is approximately fifty kilos of soiled cat litter per cat each year (in contrast, in Italy where cats are allowed outside more often, the average cat will produce only twelve kilos of waste per annum); this makes up some five per cent of Dutch refuse.

Most of the litter available to consumers is of mineral origin, made from a special kind of porous stone mined mainly in Germany, Spain, Denmark and Senegal. Such cat litter, therefore, contributes to the depletion of natural resources. The available alternatives, which are fabricated from recycled materials and which can be put in the compost bin, are growing in popularity. However, people habitually deposit ordinary litter in the special refuse bins provided for biodegradable household waste and cause great irritation for those who process the waste into compost. Like dog owners, cat owners must adequately manage their pets' excreta to prevent the refuse problem from getting even further out of hand.

Beyond the problem of dealing with pet animal excrement, sharing our homes with small animals and birds can affect our health in other respects. It is in fact interesting that so much attention has been paid to the beneficial effects of pet-keeping on human health, since this human practice can at times be a rather unhealthy one. While millions of people world-wide enjoy (or tolerate) the company of dogs and cats, there is a general lack of awareness about the *potential* health risks that these animals pose. The risk of infection of which most are aware is that which can occur through bites, most particularly from our canine companions. As discussed earlier, it has been well known since ancient times that domestic dogs can be an important agent for the transmission of rabies, although this disease has been virtually eradicated from Europe this century. Bacterial infections, such as *Pasteurella multocida*, may occur in animal bite wounds, sometimes even leading to the hospitalisation of the victim. One American study even suggests that animal bites account for some one per cent of visits to hospital emergency rooms (Schantz 1990: 15). The vast majority of bites are, however, fairly minor, though very occasionally injuries are so severe that they will require extensive plastic reconstructive surgery (Underman 1987: 196). Aside from animal bites, the toxocariasis and toxoplasmosis infections that have been discussed above present the most common threat to human health. In addition to the aforementioned diseases, humans may contract fungal dermatitis, cat scratch fever and a variety of other bacterial infections – which vary in severity – from their canine or feline friends, not to mention the allergies that they may develop to animal hair or fur.

Naturally, it is not only the common or garden varieties of pet that are responsible for, or contributors to, human illness. Rabbits, mice, guinea-pigs, hamsters, etc., for example, when bred in captivity – and providing that they are kept in sanitary conditions –

are unlikely to be too harmful to human health. However, when they are kept outside there is a danger that they will come into contact with wild rodents and birds and thus become contaminated with harmful bacteria or parasites which may be passed on to people. More exotic rodents, such as rats and gerbils, have been known to carry far nastier pathogens causing plague, Lassa fever, pseudotuberculosis to name but a few unpleasant diseases. Similarly, reptiles – such as lizards, snakes and tortoises – can carry bacteria, e.g. salmonella, which is pathogenic to humans (Stehr-Green and Schantz 1987: 6). Keeping birds may be especially detrimental to human health. Avian species are known to be the source of airborne particles – bioaerosols – which can cause allergies in humans. Moreover, it has been asserted that in households where birds are kept as pets, there is a far greater incidence of colds, throat infections, shortness of breath and flu-like symptoms, particularly if there is poor ventilation in the homes where the birds are kept. Further to this, research shows that bird-keeping may even increase the risk of children developing asthma and pregnant women spontaneously aborting. Furthermore, it has recently been suggested that bird-keeping may be a high-risk factor for human lung cancer (Holst 1991: 77).

Birds such as parrots, parakeets and budgerigars can also be responsible for chlamydia infections in humans. Psittacosis – known as ornithosis since it is also carried by birds other than parrots – is probably the most important avian zoonosis (Grimes 1987). During the nineteenth century, this disease was known to cause severe or fatal pneumonia, most particularly amongst fancy bird dealers. Today, it still largely affects those who deal with birds occupationally (Steele 1977: 17–18). Once again, the microorganism that is responsible for this disease is transmitted to humans and other birds by the aerosol in dried faeces or feather dust. Restrictions on imports of exotic birds have apparently lowered rates of infection and reduced the virulence of this respiratory disease. However, psittacosis still poses a threat to humans since there exist vast avian reservoirs that host the pathogen responsible for it not only in the caged bird population, but also amongst the farm and wild bird populations. It is not without good reason that pigeons are described as the rats of the sky, since around eighty per cent of urban pigeons are estimated to carry the infection which again can be passed on to humans through the aerosols carried in the wind (Fiennes 1978: 147). Likewise, pets can play an important role in the transmission of infectious disease to livestock. Exotic birds imported for sale as pets may, for example, carry Newcastle disease, a highly contagious and virulent disease that if transmitted to poultry can have disastrous consequences. Quarantine and import control of such birds has helped to narrow the likelihood of infection, as has domestic breeding. However, the continuing illicit trade in exotic creatures might lead to infected birds entering a country where the disease is thought to have been eradicated and farm birds becoming contaminated as a result.

While it is clear that our interactions with small animals can potentially compromise as well as benefit human health, we must not forget that conversely the close association of pet species with humans has also created new health problems for animals. In some respects, one could argue that we are killing our pets with kindness, or more to the point we are compromising their health by ignoring their basic needs and natures. Medical conditions, such as obesity and diabetes, which sometimes afflict our pampered pets are usually the direct consequence of incorrect diet, overeating and lack of exercise. Similarly, animals can become neurotic from confinement and the excessive attention of their owners (Serpell 1996). Such problems are becoming increasingly prevalent and have led to the manufacture of special diet foods for cats and dogs, in addition to the emergence of a new breed of animal doctor: the pet psychologist. Further to this, coexistence with humans and exposure to human behaviour such as smoking can increase the risk of, for instance, lung cancer for cats and dogs; such conditions are unlikely to occur when the animal is in a feral state. Likewise, increasing human dependence on and use of motorised vehicles has proved extremely hazardous to small animals causing countless injuries and fatalities amongst the pet population each year, which is ironic given that the invention of the internal combustion engine was an important factor in the rise of small-animal medicine. Finally, the effects of selective breeding and non-therapeutic surgery have had very serious consequences for pet animal health and well-being, as people have increasingly sought to transform creatures of flesh and blood into cultural objects of human desire (Swabe 1996).

It is perhaps more probable that it is the pets that more greatly suffer – quite unintentionally – from their interactions with humans than vice versa. The chances of people becoming seriously ill as a result of infection from the organisms being carried by pet animals and birds are relatively slim. We largely owe this to the efficacy of the twentieth-century veterinary regime, in addition to an increasing public concern and awareness of the necessity of taking hygienic measures in everyday life. During the course of this century, mass vaccination of pets during outbreaks of rabies (Offringa 1981: 187–8) and the institution of compulsory inoculation against rabies and passports for pets being taken across national borders has greatly contributed to the control and virtual eradication of the disease in western Europe. Furthermore, the general public has been increasingly made aware, by both veterinary professionals and the media, that if their cats and dogs are regularly wormed and their excreta disposed of properly, the possibility of humans becoming infected by the parasites which pets can carry can be greatly reduced. The same applies to birds, whose cages should be kept in a clean and well-ventilated, but not too warm, environment.

The role of the small-animal veterinary practitioner has pin this respect been largely educational, to encourage pet-owners to adopt rigorous animal management regimes, by periodically dosing their animals, keeping them in appropriate environments and being aware of the potential risks of failing to do so. The notion that pet animals may be detrimental to human health is comparatively recent, consequently there has been a lack of awareness within human medicine about the potential problems such animals might pose (Loar 1987: 17). As our intimacy and affective dependency on the species that we commonly keep as pets continues to increase, it is possible that the chances and incidences of cross-infection will also. Yet acknowledgement of the risks to human health which pet animals pose is unlikely to alter our conduct towards and relationship with them significantly. In weighing up the benefits and drawbacks of pet-keeping, it is most likely that the average (potential) pet-owner would conclude that the pleasures of sharing one's home with a cat, dog, rabbit, bird, etc., far outweigh the possible endangerment to his own or his family's health. Our present-day faith in and dependence on the veterinary profession to oversee animal health has effectively rendered such issues more or less unproblematic, lending further weight to the importance of the veterinary regime within modern society.

7

EPILOGUE

Increasing exploitation, dependency and risk

Throughout the course of history, humankind has found increasingly more effective ways of exploiting domesticated animals to service its needs and requirements. At the dawn of a new millennium, this tradition looks set to continue with a vengeance as we persist in our improvement of old, and development of new, ways in which animals can be manipulated and used to fulfil human desires. Moreover, as our exploitation of animals continues to increase, it is likely that our dependency upon them will also continue to grow, as will our potential vulnerability to them. The rapid intensification of livestock production during the twentieth century discussed earlier in this book provides perhaps the most convincing testimony to the possible consequences of such increasing exploitation of animal resources. The maximisation of production and reduction of costs through the ever-increasing concentration of larger numbers of animals in smaller spaces, use of special feeds and growth-promoting substances, etc., have greatly contributed to modern livestock production becoming an increasingly risky business; not only for the farmers who seek to make profit from their animals, but also for the public whose health can be put in jeopardy and the environment which can be seriously damaged.

In recent years, the implications of such increasing animal use for public health, animal welfare, the environment and economic fortunes have become more and more apparent, consequently becoming a firm fixture on the public, political and scientific agendas of most European nations. In particular, the impact of animal disease upon modern society has become increasingly evident during the past few years as livestock producers, the meat industry, scientists, politicians and the general public have been painfully confronted with, for example, the prospect of BSE indeed being potentially communicable to humans and numerous fatalities from food-borne infections such as *E. coli* and salmonella. This is not to mention serious outbreaks of infectious livestock disease such as classical swine fever and Newcastle disease that have put the farming economy and export markets in peril. Egged on by a highly critical mass media, the public have increasingly begun to question the nature of animal use within modern industrial society and the consequences thereof for both human health and animal welfare. However, all too often interest in this topic turns out to be fairly short-lived, and whilst a small proportion of the public may well adapt their dietary and consumer behaviour, the vast majority continue to adopt an ostrich-like approach and perpetuate the consumer demand for a constant supply of affordable animal produce of a standard quality. For this reason, and this reason alone, the intensive farming of animals remains a virtual necessity in the modern age.

The same could be said for our use of animals in general. In modern industrial society, we not only demand, but also have come to *expect*, a particular standard of living and reliable scientific solutions to our medical and technological needs. Time and again we have turned to animals to see whether they can provide the answers or living material to solve our problems. Whether it be to develop a wonder-drug to cure terminal diseases such as cancer or AIDS, or to provide the necessary organic materials to correct cardiac abnormalities, domesticated animals have continued to offer an ideal and self-replicating resource upon which we can depend in our search for solutions to human problems. Yet whilst our sensibilities towards and critique of such standard animal exploitation have clearly grown in recent decades – this being illustrated by an increasingly vocal animal rights movement – rather than decreasing our dependence upon animal resources, we appear instead to be set to intensify and diversify our exploitation yet further as we enter the twenty-first century.

Bent on extending the bounds of human knowledge and in search of new solutions to human problems, modern science has increasingly found new ways of using and modifying animals to meet human needs. In particular, the science of molecular genetics – and the biotechnological industry that has grown up alongside it – has opened up a whole host of new possibilities for the increased exploitation of animal resources. One could, in fact, say that a new scientific race is on, as scientists across the globe compete with one another to find exciting and novel ways of manipulating the animal resources they have available to them not only to create infinite future and commercial possibilities for the use of living organisms, but also to secure their own glorious place in the annals of scientific history. In this concluding chapter, I shall explore these new frontiers in animal exploitation and will contemplate what the future may hold for the role of domesticated animals in human society.

New frontiers of animal use

The scientific developments of recent years often seem like the stuff of science fiction, rather than science fact. Almost daily one can leaf through the newspapers, or turn on the television, to be confronted with news of the latest advances that will purportedly provide new hopes for the treatment of disease or the manufacture of food. Whether it be for the production of a cheaper and more effective vaccine to treat hepatitis B, or for the manufacture of a tomato that contains fish genes so that it can be successfully frozen, 'genetic engineering' – as it has been popularly dubbed – makes for good headline news because it is a topic that captures the public and scientific imagination alike. Genetics has been heralded as the science that will transform agriculture, cure diseases and conserve other species, although it could potentially also be employed to more sinister and destructive ends (Tudge 1993: ix–x). Essentially, molecular genetics is a science that explores the mechanisms of heredity. Each individual, human or animal, possesses a unique genetic 'blueprint' that makes him or her different from any other living creature. This genetic blueprint can, however, be modified. This can be achieved through a recombinant DNA technique that involves the injection of a foreign gene into an organism in order to produce specific new characteristics that in turn will also go on to be inherited by future offspring. Organisms that have been modified in such a fashion are known as 'transgenic organisms'.

The science of molecular genetics has found an increasing number of applications with regard to food-producing animals and veterinary science (Blancou 1990). In recent years, the gene mapping of farm animals has become an important tool for breeding and has been employed to localise, isolate and characterise the genes that are responsible for specific traits important to both health and production (Horzinek and van der Zijpp 1993: 84). With the development of new molecular genetic techniques that will help to isolate and identify the DNA markers that are linked to the genes responsible for economically important production traits and disease resistance, animal breeders will in the future be better equipped to single out the animals carrying the most desirable genes. Theoretically, once such genes are identified, animals may be genetically selected or engineered for disease resistance (Gogolin-Ewens *et al.* 1990). Another related application of genetic engineering is the production of more effective medical and veterinary vaccines (Wray and Woodward 1990). This may offer livestock producers a viable solution to the serious problem of enhanced infection risks that has been caused by increasingly high stocking densities. Advances in DNA recombinant technology have created the possibility for 'live carrier virus vaccines' to be developed that can be tailored to veterinary needs. It is thought that such modified live viruses will be far cheaper to manufacture and more efficient in the prevention of animal disease than existing ones (Horzinek and van der Zijpp 1993: 87–9).

Likewise, biotechnology – a term that may be generally applied to the manipulation of organisms for commercial purposes – has found important uses within animal reproduction. For many years, artificial insemination has provided the basis for the systematic genetic improvement of animals. A more recently developed reproductive technique, *in vitro* fertilisation (IVF), may possibly be employed within livestock production in the years to come. IVF involves the maturation of the egg outside the body and its fertilisation in a test tube. The embryo is then implanted into the womb of a surrogate mother. Although IVF in cattle is still in its infancy, embryo transfer is a technique that is now widely employed in livestock species and has various advantages with respect to genetic improvement, health protection and productivity (Blancou 1990: 650).

Biotechnology has also been applied to improve animal nutrition. It has been utilised at three levels: in the feed, in the digestive tract (i.e. in relation to the ruminal microflora that aids digestion) and in the physiological regulation of the animal. Genetic technology can, for example, be employed to alter rumen bacteria in order to manipulate the animal's digestive tract ecosystem. Thus far attempts to interfere with animal metabolism have met with considerable resistance (Tamminga *et al.* 1993: 169). In this respect, it is the application of an active agent, the growth hormone bovine somatotrophin (BST), to increase milk yield in cattle, that has caused perhaps the greatest consternation, raising serious questions about the lengths to which livestock producers may be willing to go in order to increase productivity. As mentioned in Chapter 5, the use of BST, which is currently produced from transgenic microbes, has been prohibited within the European Union.

One of the most controversial applications of recombinant DNA technology has been the creation of transgenic animals. The first experiments with transgenesis in mammalian species took place with animals used for laboratory experimentation. For instance, during the mid-1980s, a transgenic mouse, christened the 'oncomouse', was developed by biomedical researchers at Harvard University in their bid to understand and find a cure for breast cancer. The 'inventors' of such transgenic creatures have even gone so far as to patent their creations, leading to heated debates upon the nature of intellectual property rights and their application to living organisms (Sagoff 1996). Not surprisingly, such genetic technology has also found its way into the realms of livestock production. Since the mid-1980s, fledgling experiments with transgenesis have taken place involving food-producing animals, such as sheep, goats, pigs and cattle (Postma *et al.* 1996: 39). In the first instance, the creation of transgenic farm animals has been seen as a possible means to increase and improve agricultural productivity, to meet increasing human demands for animal produce without incurring further detriment to the environment by requisitioning extra land for agricultural production (Ward *et al.* 1990: 847–8). However, some of these transgenic experiments with food-producing species have had quite different aims. One of the prime incentives to create transgenic farm animals has been to produce substances known as biopharmaceuticals in milk. Biopharmaceuticals are substances produced by human genes that are essential to fight off disease and keep healthy. When such genes are incorporated into the DNA of other organisms, e.g. bacteria or yeast, these organisms become able to produce biopharmaceuticals beneficial to human health upon a scale that is commercially viable (Postma *et al.* 1996: 39).

A prime example of such experimentation with transgenesis and the production of biopharmaceuticals can be provided by Herman, the world's very first transgenic bull. Born in 1990 – and the result of a unique collaboration between the biotechnological company Pharming BV and a Dutch governmental research institute – Herman was the product of a fertilised egg in which the DNA had been modified to include a synthetic gene identical to the human one that controls the production of lactoferrin, a milk protein that has strong anti-microbial properties and stimulates intestinal flora to provide protection against bacterial infections (Visser 1996; Trümpler *et al.* 1989). Apart from this single gene, Herman is essentially no different to any other bull with respect to his genetic make-up. Herman was created specifically in order to sire female offspring who would inherit this foreign gene and consequently produce human lactoferrin in their milk. The first mature milk from Herman's transgenic progeny became available early in 1996 and was found to contain the appropriate lactoferrin (Postma *et al.* 1996: 42). The commercial implications of such successful biotechnological developments are potentially enormous, for they offer new possibilities for the production of pharmaceutical drugs to treat human conditions at a far lower cost. For example, Pharming, the biotech company responsible for Herman and his daughters, is currently attempting to develop a range of human health care proteins in transgenic cattle. The human lactoferrin that they have developed is intended as a component in clinical nutrition that can be used in the treatment and prevention of bacterial gastrointestinal infections in patients who have been immuno-compromised. A further planned application is in the production of speciality medical formulas for newborn and premature babies (Pharming 1995: 5). However, perhaps more importantly, the introduction of this new transgenic animal technology signifies a new role for domesticated animals within human society. It is likely that in the not-too-distant future, animals will not only continue to function as the providers of protein, but may also become living, breathing and walking 'pharmaceutical factories'.

Transgenic technology may also find other important human health applications in future years, particularly with respect to the use of animal organs for transplantation into human beings. Since organ transplant technology was first developed for the kidneys and liver and then first employed in human heart surgery by Christiaan Barnard in 1967, organ transplantation has become increasingly important in the treatment of life-threatening conditions. The continued success of surgical procedures such as kidney and heart transplantation has led to an ever-increasing demand for healthy human organs, yet – unfortunately for those awaiting such radical, though potentially life-saving, operations – there is a great shortage of suitable organs. As the population ages, it is inevitable that this demand will increase further still. In spite of numerous high profile campaigns to encourage people to carry donor codicils, the shortage of donor organs has remained critical, inspiring scientists to search for new alternatives to human organs for transplantation. Some have sought solutions in the form of artificial organs; others have begun to seriously investigate the possibilities of using animal organs for transplantation into humans (Hammer 1993).

Xenotransplantation, as such cross-species organ transplantation is known, has been heralded as a potential solution to the organ crisis, for it could provide a ready-made supply of healthy donor organs to the thousands of people who today, and in the future, will require transplant surgery. Because of the animals' genetic affinity to humans, scientists initially turned to primates – particularly baboons – in their attempts to transplant organs to humans. The very first attempt at clinical xenotransplantation in fact occurred as early as 1910 when a German medical scientist, Dr Unger, transplanted a monkey kidney into a uraemic girl. More recently, in 1992, a baboon liver was transplanted into an HIV patient who was dying of hepatitis B in the USA (Hammer 1993: 361). Primates, however, pose particularly high risks to humans with regard to the transmission of zoonotic disease, raising serious questions as to their suitability for use in xenotransplantation. The recent emergence of new highly infectious diseases such as Ebola and Marburg have further emphasised the potential role of primates as the reservoirs of viral diseases deadly to humanity (Michaels and Simmons 1994). Further to this, the use of primates in medical experimentation has become increasingly controversial due to a growing sensitivity to the semblance between humans and primate species. In recent years, calls have even been made for the great apes to be accorded equal rights to humans (Cavalieri and Singer 1993).

In view of such developments, scientific attention has instead turned to the domestic pig in the bid to produce organs suitable for human transplantation. Although more distantly related to people, the pig has already proved to be the ideal provider of insulin to treat human (and pet animal) diabetes and valves to correct heart abnormalities. Porcine organs are also approximately the same size as human ones. Moreover, given that these animals breed most prolifically, they could potentially provide a regular and reliable supply of organs for transplantation. All this being said, there are major problems that would have to be overcome before pig organs could actually be transplanted into the human body. Organ rejection is probably the greatest obstacle. This commonly occurs in the transplantation of human donor organs and is generally counteracted by the life-long usage of anti-rejection drugs by the organ recipient; in xenotransplantation rejection is likely to be hyperacute (Sykes *et al.* 1994). One of the solutions to this problem that is currently being sought by scientists is to employ transgenesis in order to genetically modify the porcine donor's organ in a way that will trick the human recipient's body into accepting it. The hearts of transgenic pigs that have been bred by researchers have already been transplanted into monkeys with some degree of success, arguably giving some indication of future possibilities for human application. The question of disease transmission through such transplant technology is also here at issue. Some porcine pathogens may indeed pose risks to human health, though it is more than likely that pigs intended for xenotransplantation will be bred to be specific-pathogen free (Michaels and Simmons 1994: 4–5). In fact, some may even be inclined to argue that the option of transplanting animal organs carries *less* disease risk than the transplantation of human donor ones. The animals used would necessarily have been genetically modified, bred and kept under strict clinical conditions; unlike the human donor who may carry all manner of diseases that may go on to infect the recipient once the organ has been transplanted.

Another recent development in the science and technology of genetics that may find its most ideal application with regard to producing transgenic animals for both transplantation and biopharmaceutical purposes is cloning. Once relegated to the realms of science fiction, cloning has today become very much a reality. In February 1996, the public and scientific world were stunned by the announcement that two genetically identical lambs, named Megan and Morag, had been born at the Roslin Institute in Scotland. These sheep had been cloned by the process of nuclear transfer from a cultured cell line, originating from different cells of the same embryo. Morag and Megan provided concrete proof of the possibility of creating animal life without the need for male sperm (Campbell *et al.* 1996). In February 1997, the even more astonishing news broke that a lamb had been cloned – by the very same scientific team – from the cells of an adult sheep. To create Dolly, as she was christened, DNA from a single cell had been taken from another sheep's udder, making her the very first mammal to have been created from the non-reproductive tissues of an adult animal (Wilmut *et al.* 1997). Dolly the sheep became a celebrity overnight and her very existence precipitated fervent debates about the ethics of cloning and its potential application to humans. A month later, hot on the hooves of this story, came the news that Australian researchers had managed to create almost five hundred genetically identical cattle clones. These were created from egg cells that had been taken from cow ovaries. At the time of writing, it remains to be seen whether these embryos can be advanced through successful pregnancies to birth (Daems 1997: 12).

The potential consequences of cloning are enormous. In the future it may well be possible to produce hundreds of copies of an adult animal. Such cloning would certainly assist the production of biopharmaceuticals in milk. Moreover, it could be feasibly used to create animals that grew faster for meat production and that were more resistant to disease; though one may imagine that a herd of identical animals may indeed be at a far greater risk of disease. Presumably, cloning could also play a role in protecting the biodiversity of species by ensuring that breeds would not die out through keeping the appropriate cells and embryos in cold storage; though at the same time it poses an enormous threat to the genetic diversity of animal species. From the point of view of both the consumer and livestock producer, cloning could theoretically ensure that meat and milk of a reliable and standard quality could be produced and sold at a standard price and would turn a standard profit. In this sense, cloning is an extremely attractive proposition for the livestock industry; as is transgenesis also – presumably these technologies will also be combined. They are, however, scientific phenomena with which many already feel extremely uncomfortable. Such technology necessarily involves direct human interference in – what is often perceived to be – the natural order and raises serious questions about the ethics and morality of such scientific enterprise. At present, national governments and scientific regulatory bodies have chosen to err very much on the side of caution when it comes to biotechnological experimentation (Cantley 1990). Often it is only when it can be proved that genetic experiments with animals can provide important benefits to humankind – as has been successfully argued for the transgenic production of lactoferrin – that they are permitted under stringent controls. Legal prohibitions on the application of such genetic technology in human beings are already firmly in place, particularly with regard to the cloning of human embryos. It remains to be seen whether either animal cloning or the production of transgenic animals will gain widespread acceptance or become commonplace in the new millennium.

Clearly, the scientific developments of recent years and the impending future present a colossal moral quagmire through which scientists, law makers and ethicists alike will be forced to wade; undoubtedly, there are also likely to be significant implications for animal welfare. However, there are also a whole host of practical problems that would have to be overcome before such technology could be successfully and safely applied. The practice of genetic engineering, for instance, carries with it an inherent risk because of pleiotropy; that is a phenomenon which occurs when a gene that does one specific thing may have other, possibly unrelated, effects upon or could interfere with the behaviour of other genes (Tudge 1993: 243). One of the major and commonly espoused objections to the genetic technology that has been developed in recent years is that it necessarily involves the deliberate and wholesale interference with 'nature's design'. Further to this, the idea of genetically modifying other life forms has also met with considerable hostility for it reeks of eugenics; the implications of which are still fresh in our collective memory from the darker events of the twentieth century. History has already taught us that the calculated 'improvement' of humans can be a highly dangerous business with the most sinister of consequences. Yet leaving the issue of the application of genetic technology to humans aside and focusing upon animals alone, it is pertinent to consider just how well grounded our objections to and fears of the genetic modification of animals actually are.

Although the genetic technology of recent times has often been portrayed as an extremely new and outlandish development, the fact remains that there is – at least in principle – very little new about it; most certainly as far as animals are concerned. The genetic modification of animals can logically be viewed as an extension, or rather a continuation of the process of domestication and selective breeding that has already been going on for the past 10,000 or so years. As this book has sought to illustrate, for thousands of years, humankind has actively attempted – in ever-increasingly successful measures – to alter and improve the behaviour, physical appearance and productivity of animals in order to service its needs. Whether it be to produce a more tractable animal or one that will produce more milk or larger calves, animals have persistently been deliberately and selectively bred to achieve highly specific ends. In this sense, people have been practising the art of 'genetic engineering' since animals were first domesticated. Traditionally, new varieties of animal species have been produced by cross-breeding. Until very recently, breeders had no detailed knowledge of the genetic mechanisms involved in producing such new varieties. Animal husbandry was a purely empirically based occupation. Farmers gradually learned that if, for example, cattle that produced a high milk yield were bred with other high-milk-yielding cattle, they would produce offspring that would go on to produce even more milk. This kind of genetic manipulation is, however, far from an exact science. Moreover, such selective breeding can take an extremely long time before it produces the desirable result. Recombinant DNA technology has expedited this process, for it has provided the means by which the genetic make-up of animals can be modified in order to produce specific traits that – by traditional means – would have taken many generations to introduce, or would never have occurred at all since they involve the insertion of DNA foreign to the recipient animal.

Likewise, although many tend to balk at the mention of it, there is little new about biotechnology. Biotechnology can essentially be defined as 'the application of scientific and engineering principles to the processing of materials by biological agents to produce goods and services' (Wray and Woodward 1990: 779). Whilst this may sound like a new-fangled idea, the fact remains that humankind has been using biotechnological techniques for many thousands of years in order to manufacture products such as beer, wine and bread. To make such products, microorganisms have been routinely and deliberately manipulated for highly specific ends. The role of yeast in bread baking is perhaps the best example of this. Again, it has been the development of recombinant DNA technology that has increased the capabilities of biotechnological production, rendering it an important and efficient technique for the future. As has already been suggested, it is likely that biotechnology will play an increasingly important role in veterinary medical science, particularly with respect to the improvement of animal health and nutrition, the production of veterinary vaccines and prevention of animal disease. As a corollary to this, biotechnology may also be crucial to the maintenance of public health as it may contribute greatly to the control of zoonotic disease (Callis *et al.* 1989).

There are, however, good reasons why we should be cautious about the application of recombinant DNA technology to domesticated animals. Selective breeding, in the traditional fashion, has already proved to have had serious consequences for animal health and welfare. Take, for example, the current state of broiler chickens and turkeys that have been bred to grow so fast and produce such grossly enlarged breast muscle tissue that their legs become crippled; or the double-muscled Belgian Blue calves that necessarily have to be born by caesarean section. Such breeding practices have been developed in the constant bid to increase productivity to meet consumer demands and to produce higher profits, generally at the expense of animal well-being. But, as Chapter 6 illustrated, it is not only the food-producing species that have fallen foul to irresponsible breeding practices. The health and well-being of pet animals have also been compromised severely through breeders' continued attempts to produce new varieties and to emphasise specific animal characteristics. One could argue that the application of genetic technology could plausibly solve many of the problems created by both intensive farming practices and pet-keeping. For example, it may in the future be possible to create a race of hornless cattle, thus obviating the need for dehorning altogether. Likewise, transgenic chickens might be produced that lack nerves to their beaks and could thus be debeaked without causing them any pain. Whilst such developments may indeed be possible, they will nonetheless do nothing to improve the general conditions in which intensively farmed livestock live and are bred (Tudge 1993: 245). Similarly, transgenic cats could be produced without claws and dogs with modified vocal cords for the convenience of their human owners.

It remains to be seen whether the genetic modification of animals will create serious new problems with regard to animal welfare. The application of recombinant DNA technology to animals is so recent that it cannot yet be said with any great certainty whether, for example, the inclusion of a single human gene to cattle in order to produce biopharmaceuticals will endanger animal health and well-being in any fashion. Nor for that matter whether it may affect the health of humans who consume such genetically modified milk or its pharmaceutical derivatives. It is likely that such cattle will essentially continue to function just as and be treated like any other dairy animal. In that sense, transgenesis may change little with regard to how animals will live within human society. Creating transgenic pigs (and possibly other species also) for xenotransplantation, on the other hand, will most likely entail that the animals be kept in extremely sterile, clinical environments that are a far cry from the conditions, for better or worse, that they now experience. What is, however, clear is that with the introduction of genetic engineering, our manipulation and exploitation of animals has entered a brand new phase. The production of new animal varieties can now take place over the course of one single generation, rather than many. Moreover, and perhaps more importantly, recombinant DNA technology means that animals can be modified using genetic material that is completely alien to the recipient animal species. Needless to say, this signifies a crucial new development in the age-old practice of animal husbandry. It remains to be seen to what extent the practice of genetic engineering will be continued and commercially employed, or whether this will be deemed ethically and biologically unacceptable.

Concluding remarks

As the new millennium approaches, it is clear that the role of domesticated animals in human society is continuing to diversify, rather than diminish. Whilst it appears that many people are becoming more sensitive to the lot and rights of other animals, humanity as a whole seems to be perpetuating the tacit belief that animals may be exploited as a natural resource. In this respect, the message of this book is rather bleak for those who seek to reduce or rid the world of animal exploitation. For the foreseeable future, this is unlikely to happen; though it does not necessarily exclude the possibility that animals could well be treated in a more humane fashion whilst being used by humankind. A world where animal flesh is no longer eaten, nor animals exploited for human ends in any way, remains steadfastly within the realms of fantasy and science fiction. The utopian vision of *Star Trek* where humanity has attained the pinnacle of civilisation by no longer breeding and killing animals for food, instead obtaining its nutrients and raw materials through synthetic replication, is far removed from the stark realities of the twentieth – and probably twenty-first – century. Contrary to what many may hope, the human exploitation of animals has greatly increased and looks set to increase still further in the years to come as new uses for animals are dreamt up along with the new technologies that can achieve them.

The final question remains of just what these developments will entail for the veterinary regime. It seems likely that as the frontiers of animal exploitation continue to expand, so will the importance of veterinary medical science to society also. Veterinary expertise has thus far been crucial to the development of transgenic animals for the production of biopharmaceuticals and xenotransplantation. The close interaction between veterinarians and scientists from other academic spheres will presumably continue as such technologies are further refined or expanded. Scientific developments seem likely to require that in the future veterinarians will be obliged to be complicit in the activities of the biotechnologists, as much as they have become in the activities of the livestock industry during the post-war period. If biotechnology turns out to offer all that it today seems to promise, then it seems certain that the efficacy of the veterinary regime will improve further still. The prospect of new and more effective vaccines to combat animal disease and the improvement of animal nutrition have great implications for both the health and well-being of animals and public health. If the damage caused by animal disease is reduced and the methods of controlling it become cheaper, the consumer will undoubtedly also reap the benefits of veterinary advances through being able to buy safer, cheaper and better quality animal produce. However, at present, many consumers are sceptical about the advantages that genetic technology purportedly offers and the impact that it will have upon their lives. Likewise, policy-makers and legislators have responded cautiously to recent scientific advances and have been keen to exercise their regulatory powers upon the burgeoning biotechnological industry. In this respect, as we enter the twenty-first century, the state is likely to tighten its grip still further and continue its imposition of the veterinary regime with increased vigour, particularly within an international framework. Throughout the course of the late twentieth century, the importance of an effective veterinary regime has become increasingly evident. Calamities such as the recent BSE crisis have explicitly highlighted the potential consequences of our increased exploitation of animals and the necessity of intensifying measures for animal disease control. As the new millennium dawns, it seems more than likely the burden of beasts for human society will continue to be a heavy one.

APPENDIX

Table 2 Cattle by-products

Principal by-products obtained from cattle	*Finished by-products prepared by packer*	*By-products manufactured after leaving packers*
Hide (including cured hide, tail hair, body hair, lar hair, hide trimmings and fat)	Glue Tallow	Leather (saddlery, shoes, belts, etc.) Upholstery Brushes Felting Plaster
Fats (including edible oleo fat and inedible tallow fat)	Bakery products (margarine, shortening) Animal feed Stearine & Glycerine (soap)	Industrial products
Head (including bones, horns, brains, tongue, head & cheek meat, ox lips and palates)	Bone meal Sausages Animal feed	Protective colloid plaster retarder
Feet (including dew claws, sinews, bones and hooves)	Tallow, glue Bone meal Animal feed Fertiliser	Protective colloid plaster retarder
Blood (fresh and dried)	Sausages Plasma, aiomin, fibrin Plant food Animal feed	Textile sizing Weatherproof glue Pharmaceutical uses

Table 2 (cont.)

Principal by-products obtained from cattle	*Finished by-products prepared by packer*	*By-products manufactured after leaving packers*
Casings (including bladder & intestines)	Sausage casings Cheese containers Tallow Animal feed	Parchment
Miscellaneous (including heart, liver, sweetbread, tail, kidneys, tripe, glands and gall bag)	Sausage Animal feed	Medical and drug uses Perfume

Source: Based on Kotula (1991: 298–9). It is worth noting that since the emergence of BSE, bans on the usage of specified offals have been introduced in order to prevent the disease-causing agent from entering the food chain.

Table 3 Pig by-products

Principal by-products obtained from pigs	*Finished by-products prepared by packer*	*By-products manufactured after leaving packer*
Skin (including bristles, hair and pork skin)	Glue Gelatine	Brushes Felting, upholstering, plaster retardant, insulation Leather goods Fish bait
Fats (including lean fat, edible killing fats, cutting fats and inedible fats)	Lard Margarine Animal feed Fatty acids (red oil, stearic acid, glycerine, pitch) Soap	Salves Cosmetics Soap Carbon paper Textile lubricants Candles Tyres Roofing and paving compounds Medicine Explosives Moisture retainer Moulds Defoamers Tanning Cleaning emulsions Lubricating grease
Casings (including stomach and bladder)	Sausage containers Tripe Grease Animal feed	Pepsin
Blood	Fertiliser Animal feed Sausage	
Gall		Pharmaceutical uses

Table 3 (cont.)

Principal by-products obtained from pigs	*Finished by-products prepared by packer*	*By-products manufactured after leaving packer*
Glands (including pancreas, ovaries, thyroid, pituitary and suprarenal)		Pharmaceutical uses
Head (including tongue, ears, lips, snout, cheek and head meat, brain and bones)	Sausage Lard Glue Fertiliser Animal feed	
Miscellaneous (including feet, tail, heart, liver, lungs and kidneys)	Lard Glue Sausage Animal feed	Liver extract pharmaceutics

Source: Based on Kotula (1991: 300–1).

Table 4 Lamb by-products

Principal by-products obtained from lambs	*Finished by-products prepared by packer*	*By-products manufactured after leaving packer*
Head (including brains, tongue, cheek and head, bones and inedible fats)	Sausage Glue Glycerine Soap	Cosmetics Polish base Soaps
Pelt (including pulled wool, skin after removal of fleece, trimmings, tanned short wool pelt)	Clean fleece Lanolin	Clothing Knitting yarns Upholstery Blankets Cosmetics
Trotters	Glue Tallow Soap Fertiliser Animal feed	Soap Fertiliser Animal feed
Fats (edible and inedible)	Tallow Stearine Glycerine Soap	Leather dressing Pharmaceutical uses Anti-freeze Paints Cellophane Liquid soap Medicinal preparations Cosmetics Polish base
Blood (fresh and dried)	Sausage Blood flour Blood meal Animal feed	Albumin – weatherproof glue Serum Pharmaceutical uses
Casings	Sausage containers	Plaster retardant Strings of musical instruments Tennis racquets Surgical catgut Pharmaceutical uses

Table 4 (cont.)

Principal by-products obtained from lambs	*Finished by-products prepared by packer*	*By-products manufactured after leaving packer*
Fancy meats (including heart, liver, sweetbreads, kidneys, stomach)	Sausage	Animal feed
Glands (including pituitary, thyroid, ovaries, pancreas and superarenal)		Pharmaceutical uses

Source: Based on Kotula (1991: 302–3).

NOTES

1 INTRODUCTION

1 Indeed, as anthropologist Marvin Harris has astutely observed, no major world religion has ever urged its followers to adopt the practice of veganism, nor for that matter have they entirely prohibited the consumption of eggs and animal flesh from the diets of ordinary people (Harris 1985a: 23).

2 There are often either synthetically produced or vegetable-derived alternatives to animal by-products available to manufacturers. Cheese, for example, can be produced using a vegetable rennet, just as glycerine can be obtained from vegetable sources. However, particularly where E numbers are concerned, it is not always clear whether they are of animal, vegetable or synthetic origin. Moreover, the consumer has no direct way of telling when they purchase a product.

3 Our relationship with wild and laboratory animals, fish and insects has been excluded from the discussion, although these categories will be referred to when directly relevant to the matter at hand.

4 Admittedly, my explorations into veterinary history have indeed been restricted somewhat by the limitations of language. German veterinary historical literature is reportedly far more reliable and better written than the texts that many English-language authors have produced. Throughout my research, one text, *Geschichte der Tiermedizin: 5000 Jahre Tierheilkunde* (von den Driesch 1989), has been consistently recommended to me. Unfortunately, as interesting and comprehensive as this volume looks, my German is far too poor to have derived any benefit from it. A translation of this text would certainly not go amiss. Further to this, the numerous French- and German-language dissertations that have been written in the field of veterinary history should not be overlooked. A recent selection of these were reviewed in *Argos*, the Dutch journal for veterinary history (1997: 16: 257–8). See also Fischer (1988: 206–9) for extensive references to German Ph.D. dissertations that have specifically dealt with aspects of ancient veterinary medicine.

2 DOMESTICATION, DEPENDENCY AND DISEASE

1 Eating foods of plant origin would also have been potentially hazardous to our ancestors. Some species of plant and the fruits they bear can be toxic, moreover plants can also carry fungi which can cause illness in both humans and other animals.

2 Three important species – the camel, llama and alpaca – have deliberately been omitted from this list of domesticates since they do not play a significant role in European society. The camel – originating in southern Arabia – and these South American camelid species are all believed to have been domesticated around 3000 BC. The camel became a valuable animal for transportation in the desert regions of Arabia and North Africa; similarly, the llama became a beast of burden and – like its close relative the alpaca – it has been exploited by Andean peoples for its wool, meat, hide and dung for centuries.

3 In this sense, many of the species such as lions, tigers, rhinoceroses, bears, etc., which we consider to be quintessentially wild, often live almost exclusively in culturally controlled environments. National parks, established to preserve endangered indigenous animal species, are as much social institutions as zoos, yet we do not conventionally think of their habitats being socially constructed. The mortal danger presented by animal species seems to determine our perception of their degree of wildness and their proximity to human society is gauged by their potential usefulness to humankind. The predicament of deer in western Europe provides a good illustration of this; these animals live on the fringes of the wild and the tame. They seldom live outside culturally controlled environments, are regularly hunted for food or sport, but are regarded with affection by many. They are not domesticated, but can they really still be considered wild?

3 ANIMALS, DISEASE AND HUMAN SOCIAL LIFE

1 Schwabe has observed that the ankh, one of the oldest and most prominent Egyptian divine symbols signifying life, bears striking resemblance to the bull's thoracic vertebra (Schwabe 1986: 257).

2 Alexander the Great successfully adapted the military method of the phalanx and applied it to cavalry warfare. This human–horse configuration presented a formidable force to his enemies (McNeill 1963: 243n).

3 The Middle Ages is here understood as the period spanning from around AD 400 to AD 1400. For an excellent and extensive overview of changing human–animal relations during this period, I refer the reader to Salisbury (1994).

4 Indeed, as Keith Thomas points out, the animal population was, in the past, far larger than the human one. In early sixteenth-century England, there were approximately three sheep to every one person; in modern times this ratio has been reversed (Thomas 1983: 94).

5 Other parasitic infections, such as dracontiasis, are also known to have afflicted the early Egyptians with pain and disability. Adamson (1988)

suggests that the guineaworm, which causes this disease, may have been introduced by traders who brought infected primates from central Africa. Apes were sacred animals to the Egyptians, representing the god Thoth, and were kept by priests in temples or as tame pets in private homes. Dogs were also a likely reservoir for dracontiasis; the early Egyptians' close association with them created possibilities for transmission between species (Adamson 1988: 207).

6 For a detailed chronological account of the history of these animal plagues and their impact on European agricultural society, I refer the reader to Fleming (1871).

4 THE UNFOLDING VETERINARY REGIME

1 It is in fact now believed that when St. Bel died of an acute infection, a mere year after the London Veterinary College opened, he had actually been suffering from glanders, probably transmitted from infected horses stabled at the college. Ironically, it appears that the French professor neither believed that the disease could be transmitted by inoculation in animals, nor did he suspect that it was transmissible to humans. Nearly two decades were to pass before it was realised that glanders could indeed be communicated to people, and cases of human glanders came to be identified by both military and civil surgeons across Europe (Wilkinson 1992: 118–21).

2 It is interesting to note that unlike in other European nations, where the practice of veterinary medicine eventually became the sole preserve of the qualified veterinary school graduate, in the Netherlands other individuals continue, to this day, to provide specific veterinary services. Specialist para-veterinarians, such as castrators, cattle 'midwives' and 'keurmeesters' (lay meat inspectors), operate within Dutch society, although they too must have received adequate training and certification from state-recognised institutions; these people are, however, today increasingly few and far between.

3 Such scathing public remarks are quite typical of the ideological battles between contagionists and anti-contagionists that were being fought at this time, particularly with regard to public health matters (Goudsblom 1986; Worboys 1992).

5 THE INTENSIFICATION OF LIVESTOCK PRODUCTION

1 Today, largely as a consequence of selective breeding, calves will often weigh this much at birth.

2 One of the reasons why poultry has become so popular with the modern consumer is that, compared with red meat products, it is so quick and easy to prepare.

3 The resistance of infective agents to and ineffectiveness of sterilisation has also been illustrated by the case of Bovine Spongiform Encephalopathy (BSE). The emergence of BSE has been attributed to the supplementary feed – given to cattle to increase milk yield – which

contained the inadequately sterilised brains of sheep infected with scrapie (Anderson *et al*. 1996).

4 It should be noted that tuberculosis, brucellosis and trichinosis no longer pose a threat to public health in western Europe. These diseases do, however, persist in other parts of the globe.

5 Just how unfamiliar the average consumer is with modern livestock production methods can be illustrated by the kind of shock reaction and public outcry that occurs when images of such farms are shown during news broadcasts and documentaries. The fervent public response to the news footage of intensive pig production in the Netherlands that was televised in relation to the 1997 outbreak of classical swine fever provides a good example of this.

6 Whilst the need for animal disease control may have been firmly embedded in the habitus of livestock producers, it does not preclude the possibility that farmers will deliberately choose to go against veterinary advice or legislation for animal disease control, putting the health of their own and other people's livestock and/or public health at risk. For example, failures to comply with and attempts to circumvent animal transport restrictions during the early phases of the recent Dutch classical swine fever epidemic are believed to have contributed to the spread of the disease.

7 Anthrax spores, for example, can survive for fifty years (or more in soil) even when they are exposed to sunlight or dry air which usually destroy other dangerous disease-producing organisms, e.g. brucella, in a matter of days (Winkler 1982: 12).

8 It can, however, also be argued that the practice of livestock keeping greatly contributes to these world food shortages. Many of the cattle herds that supply the Western consumer with abundant supplies of meat are grain-fed. This can be seen as a terrible waste of valuable resources, since this grain could be used to feed people, rather than animals. As Peter Singer puts it, 'the heavy emphasis in affluent nations on rearing animals for food wastes several times as much food as it produces' (Singer 1990: vii). He suggests that if we stopped rearing and killing animals for food, and distributed grain reserves more equally, starvation and malnutrition would be eliminated. How feasible redistribution of these granular resources amongst the Third World populations would be is another matter, as is the affluent nations ceasing livestock production.

9 The above comments upon the identification and registration of individual animals are based on the current situation in the Netherlands. In Great Britain, for example, such a system of tagging cattle does not yet exist. The need for such a system whereby individual animals can, at least in principle, be traced, became evident during the recent BSE epidemic.

10 Whilst it is true to say that livestock and animal tissue are subject to strict veterinary control, modern livestock markets and abattoirs are increasingly becoming the hotbeds of bacterial contamination. Conveyor-belt-style abattoirs that handle large numbers of live animals or carcasses using the same equipment enhance the risk of cross-contamination. Failure to adhere to hygienic standards and the speed

at which 'line processing' of animals operates provide greater opportunities for bacteria to flourish (cf. Johnson 1991: 86).

11 Though in saying this, it is indeed often the consumer who is to blame. Food of animal origin is frequently improperly handled, unsuitably stored and inadequately cooked by people, leading to outbreaks of food poisoning which might have otherwise been avoided.

6 PANDERING TO PETS

1 This in itself is noteworthy for it is widely thought that tail-docking originated as a practical measure to allow working dogs to perform their tasks more efficiently. Although amputating dogs' tails was undoubtedly of some functional benefit in some working breeds, it may well be possible that this custom has its origins in beliefs about rabies. Whatever the case, it is nonetheless interesting that this practice has become embedded in notions of how breeds should appear; both the functional aspects of tail-docking and notions of rabies prevention having been lost to history.

2 This is, of course, not to mention the waste problem created by the hundreds of thousands of empty pet food tins discarded each year.

BIBLIOGRAPHY

Ackerknecht, E.H. and Fischer-Homberger, E. (1977) 'Five Made it – One not: The Rise of Medical Craftsmen to Academic Status During the 19th Century'. *Clio Medica.* 12: 4, pp.255– 67.

Adamson, P.B. (1976) 'Schistosomiasis in Antiquity'. *Medical History*. 20, pp.176–88.

——(1988) 'Dracontiasis in Antiquity'. *Medical History*. 32, pp.204–9.

——(1989) 'Diseases Associated with Man and Pig in the Ancient Near East'. *Historia Medicinae Veterinariae*. 14: 4, pp.104–10.

Albertus Magnus (1987) *Man and the Beasts (De Animalibus: Books 22–6)* [Translated by Scanlan, J.J.: Mediaeval and Renaissance Texts and Studies]. Binghamton: New York.

Anderson, B.K., Hart, B.L. and Hart, A.L. (eds) (1984) *The Pet Connection: Its Influence on Our Health and Quality of Life*. Minneapolis: University of Minnesota Press.

Anderson, J.K. (1961) *Ancient Greek Horsemanship*. Berkeley: University of California Press.

Anderson, R.M., Donnelly, C.A., Ferguson, N.M., Woolhouse, M.E.J., Watt, C.J., Udy, H.J., Mawhinney, S., Dunstan, S.P., Southwood, T.R.E., Wilesmith, J.M., Ryan, J.B.M., Hoinville, L.J., Hillerton, J.E., Austin, A.R. and Wells, G.A.H. (1996) 'Transmission Dynamics and Epidemiology of BSE in British Cattle'. *Nature*. 382, pp.779–88.

Arluke, A. and Sanders, C.R. (1996) *Regarding Animals*. Philadelphia: Temple University Press.

Ash, E.C. (1927) *Dogs: Their History and Development*. New York: Benjamin Blom.

Azzaroli, A. (1985) *An Early History of Horsemanship*. Leiden: Brill & Backuys.

Baker, J. and Brothwell, D. (1980) *Animal Diseases in Archaeology*. London: Academic Press.

Baker, S. (1993) *Picturing the Beast: Animals, Identity and Representation*. Manchester: Manchester University Press.

Ballarini, G. and Ferrando, R. (1988) 'Naissance des Écoles Vétérinaires'. *Recueil de Médecine Vétérinaire*. 168: 1, pp.11–16.

Barclay, H.B. (1980) *The Role of the Horse in Man's Culture*. London: J.A. Allen.

Barker, G. (1985) *Prehistoric Farming in Europe*. Cambridge: Cambridge University Press.

Bieleman, J. (1992) *Geschiedenis van de Landbouw in Nederland 1500–1950*. Amsterdam: Boom.

Bisseru, B. (1967) *Diseases of Man Acquired from His Pets*. London: William Heinemann.

Blaine, D.P. (1800) *A Concise Description of Distemper in Dogs, With an Account of the Discovery of an Efficacious Remedy for It.*

——(1817) *Canine Pathology*. London: Boosey.

Blaisdell, J.D. (1994) 'The Curse of the Pharaohs: Anthrax in Ancient Egypt'. *Argos: Bulletin van het Veterinair Historisch Genootschap*. 10, pp. 311–14.

Blake, N.F. (1980) *The Canterbury Tales by Geoffrey Chaucer*. (Edited from the Hengwrt Manuscript.) London: Edward Arnold.

Blancou, J. (1990) 'Utilisation and Control of Biotechnological Procedures in Veterinary Science'. *Revue Scientifique et Technique de l'Office International des Epizooties*. 9: 3, pp.641–59.

——(1994) 'Early Methods for the Surveillance and Control of Glanders in Europe'. *Revue Scientifique et Technique de l'Office International des Epizooties.* 13: 2, pp.545–58.

Blood, D.C. (1994) *Pocket Companion to Veterinary Medicine*. London: Baillière Tindall.

Bodson, L. (1994) 'Ancient Views on Pests and Parasites of Livestock'. *Argos: Bulletin van het Veterinair Historisch Genootschap*. 10, pp. 303–10.

——(1996) 'Veterinary Medicine'. In Hornblower, S. and Spawforth, A. (eds) *The Oxford Classical Dictionary*. Oxford: Oxford University Press. pp. 1592–3.

Bökönyi, S. (1969) 'Archaeological Problems and Methods of Recognizing Animal Domestication'. In Ucko, P.J. and Dimbleby, G.W. (eds) *The Domestication and Exploitation of Plants and Animals*. London: Duckworth. pp. 219–29.

——(1989) 'Definitions of Animal Domestication'. In Clutton-Brock, J. (ed.) *The Walking Larder: Patterns of Domestication, Pastoralism, and Predation*. London: Unwin Hyman. pp.22–7.

Bonner, J. (1997) 'Hooked on Drugs'. *New Scientist*. 18 January 1997, pp. 24–7.

Boor-van der Putten, I.M.E. (1986) *75 Jaar Geneeskunde van Gezelschapsdieren in Nederland*. Utrecht: Faculteit Diergeneeskunde.

——(1990) 'De Geneeskunde van de Hond in de Veertiende Eeuw volgens de *Livre de Chasse* van Gaston Phebus'. *Argos: Bulletin van het Veterinair Historisch Genootschap*. Speciale Uitgave, pp.60–7.

Bourdieu, P. (1984) *Distinction: A Social Critique of the Judgement of Taste*. London: Routledge & Kegan Paul.

Bouw, J. (1991) 'Domesticatie'. *Argos: Bulletin van het Veterinair Historisch Genootschap*. Speciale Uitgave, pp.23–8.

Bowler, J. (1990) *The Vegetarian Handbook* (18th edition). Altrincham: The Vegetarian Society UK.

Bracken, H. (1738) *Farriery Improv'd*. London: Printed for J.Clarke.

Brander, G.C. and Ellis, P.R. (1977) *The Control of Disease*. London: Baillière Tindall.

Brock, T.D. (1961) *Milestones in Microbiology*. London: Prentice-Hall.

——(1988) *Robert Koch: A Life in Medicine and Bacteriology*. Berlin: Springer-Verlag.

Broom, D.M. and Johnson, K.G. (1993) *Stress and Animal Welfare*. London: Chapman & Hall.

Brothwell, D.R. (1991) 'On Zoonoses and their Relevance to Paleopathology'. In Ortner, D.J. and Aufderheide, A.C. (eds) *Human Paleopathology: Current Syntheses and Future Opinions*. Washington: Smithsonian Institution Press. pp. 18–22.

Browne, W. (1620) *Browne his Fiftie Yeares Practice*. London: Printed by Nicholas Oakes.

——(1624) *The Horse-mans Honour, Or, the Beautie of Horsemanship*. London: Printed by Nicholas Oakes.

Budiansky, S. (1992) *The Covenant of the Wild: Why Animals Chose Domestication*. London: Weidenfeld & Nicolson.

Burnet, M. and White, D.O. (1972) *Natural History of Disease* (Fourth edition). Cambridge: Cambridge University Press.

Caius, J. (1576) *Of Englishe Dogges, the Diversities, the Names, the Natures and the Properties*. (Newly drawne into English by Abraham Fleming, student.) London: Richard Johnes.

Callis, J., Bachrach, H., Bittle, J., Dalrymple, J., Gamble, R., Glosser, J., Murphy, F., Thiermann, A. and Thompson, S. (1989) 'Biotechnology and its Public Health Implications in Zoonotic Diseases'. In Animal Production and Health Division, FAO *Biotechnology and Livestock Production*. New York: Plenum Press. pp.377–400.

Campbell, K.H.S., McWhir, J., Ritchie, W.A. and Wilmut, I. (1996) 'Sheep Cloned by a Nuclear Transfer from a Cultured Cell Line'. *Nature*. 380, pp. 60–66.

Cantley, M.F. (1990) 'Regulatory Aspects of Biotechnology in Europe, with Particular Reference to Veterinary Science'. *Revue Scientifique et Technique de l'Office International des Epizooties*. 9: 3, pp. 659–713.

Cavalieri, P. and Singer, P. (1993) *Great Ape Project: Equality beyond Humanity*. London: Fourth Estate.

Centraal Bureau voor Statistiek (CBS) (1996) *Agriculture Census 1996*. Voorburg, Heerlen: Statistics Netherlands.

Charnock Bradley, O. (1923) *History of the Edinburgh Veterinary College*. Edinburgh: Edinburgh University Library.

Clayton, B. (188?) *Dogs: How to Breed and Treat, in Health and Disease*. London: Dean & Son.

Clutton-Brock, J. (1987) *A Natural History of Domesticated Mammals*. Cambridge: Cambridge University Press.

——(1988) *The British Museum Book of Cats: Ancient and Modern*. London: British Museum

——(1989) 'Introduction to Domestication'. In Clutton-Brock, J. (ed.) *The Walking Larder: Patterns of Domestication, Pastoralism, and Predation*. London: Unwin Hyman. pp. 7–9.

——(1992) *Horse Power*. Cambridge, MA: Harvard University Press.

——(1994) 'The Unnatural World: Behavioural Aspects of Humans and Animals in the Process of Domestication'. In Manning, A. and Serpell, J. (eds) *Animals and Human Society: Changing Perspectives*. London: Routledge. pp. 36–58.

Cockburn, A. (1963) *The Evolution and Eradication of Infectious Diseases*. Baltimore: Johns Hopkins Press.

Cohen, M.N. (1977) *The Food Crisis in Prehistory: Overpopulation and the Origins of Agriculture*. New Haven: Yale University Press.

Cohen, M.N. and Armelagos, G.J. (1984) 'Editors' Summation'. In Cohen, M.N. and Armelagos, G.J. (eds) *Paleopathology at the Origins of Agriculture*. New York: Academic Press. pp. 585–601.

Columella, L.J.M. (1745) *Of Husbandry.*(Translated into English.) London: A. Millar.

Cotchin, E. (1990) *The Royal Veterinary College London: A Bicentenary History*. Buckingham: Barracuda.

Crosby, A.W. (1994) *Germs, Seeds and Animals: Studies in Ecological History*. New York: M.E. Sharpe.

CSS Report (1988) *Companion Animals in Society*. Oxford: Oxford University Press.

Cunningham, W. (1976) 'The Work of Two Scottish Medical Graduates in the Control of Woolsorters' Disease' (The Scottish Society of the History of Medicine: Report of Proceedings 1974–75). *Medical History*. 20, pp.169–72.

CVL (1994) *CVL 100 years: 1894–1994 Working for Animal Health*. Weybridge, Surrey: CVL.

D'Arcy Thompson, R. (1974) *The Remarkable Gamgees: A Story of Achievement*. Edinburgh: Ramsey Head Press.

Daems, W. (1997) 'Dolly, het Schaap dat uit een Uier Kwam'. *EOS Magazine: Wetenschap en Technologie voor de Mens*. pp.9–13.

Davids, K. (1989) *Dieren en Nederlanders: Zeven Eeuwen van Lief en Leed*. Utrecht: Mattrijs.

Davis, S.J.M. (1987) *The Archaeology of Animals*. London: B.T. Batsford.

Dekkers, M. (1992) *Lief Dier: Over Bestialiteit*. Amsterdam: Uitgeverij Contact.

Diamond, J. (1997) *Guns, Germs and Steel*. London: Jonathan Cape.

Dixon, K.R. and Southern, P. (1992) *The Roman Cavalry: From the First to the Third Century AD*. London: B.T. Batsford.

Dolan, T.M. (1879) *The Nature and Treatment of Rabies or Hydrophobia*. London; Baillière, Tindall & Cox.

Douglas, M. (1966) *Purity and Danger*. London: Routledge & Kegan Paul.

Doyen-Higuet, A-M. (1984) 'The *Hippiatrica* and Byzantine Veterinary Medicine'. In Scarborough, J. (ed.) *Symposium on Byzantine Medicine*. Washington: Dumbarton Oaks Papers. pp.109–20.

Driesch, A. von den (1989) *Geschichte der Tiermedizin: 5000 Jahre Tierheilkunde*. Munich: Callwey.

Dubey, J.P. and Beattie, C.P. (1988) *Toxoplasmosis of Animals and Man*. Boca Raton, Florida: CRC Press.

Ducos, P. (1989) 'Defining Domestication: A Clarification'. In Clutton-Brock, J. (ed.) *The Walking Larder: Patterns of Domestication, Pastoralism, and Predation*. London: Unwin Hyman. pp.28–30.

Dunlop, R. and Williams, D. (1996) *Veterinary Medicine: An Illustrated History*. St Louis: Mosby.

'E.H.' (1865) *The Cattle Plague of 1865 and its Cure*. London: Epps & Co.

El-Ahraf, A. and Willis, W.V. (1996) *Management of Animal Waste: Environmental Health Problems and Technological Solutions*. Westport, Connecticut: Praeger.

Elias, N. (1994) *The Civilising Process*. (Translated by Jephcott, E. German original published 1939.) Oxford: Blackwell.

Endenburg, N. (1991) *Animals as Companions: Demographic, Motivational and Ethical Aspects of Companion Animal Ownership*. Ph.D. Thesis. Rijksuniversiteit Utrecht.

Endenburg, N. and Baarda, B. (1995) 'The Role of Pets in Enhancing Human Well-being: Effects on Child Development'. In Robinson, I. (ed.) *The Waltham Book of Human–Animal Interaction: Benefits and Responsibilities of Pet-Ownership*. Oxford: Pergamon. pp.7–18.

Fiddes, N. (1991) *Meat: A Natural Symbol*. London: Routledge.

Fiennes, R.N.T-W. (1978) *Zoonoses and the Origins and Ecology of Human Disease*. London: Academic Press.

Fischer, K-D. (1988) 'Ancient Veterinary Medicine: A Survey of Greek and Latin Sources and some Recent Scholarship'. *Medizinhistorisches Journal*. 23, pp.191–209.

Fisher, J. R. (1979/80) 'Professor Gamgee and the Farmers'. *Veterinary History*. 1: 2, pp.47–63.

——(1993) 'Not Quite a Profession: The Aspirations of Veterinary Surgeons in England in the Mid-Nineteenth Century'. *Historical Research*. 66, pp.284–302.

——(1995) 'The European Enlightenment, Political Economy and the Origins of the Veterinary Profession in Britain'. *Argos: Bulletin van het Veterinair Historisch Genootschap*. 12, pp.45–51.

——(1997) 'Of Plagues and Veterinarians: BSE in Historical Perspective'. *Argos: Bulletin van het Veterinair Historisch Genootschap*. 16, pp.225–33.

Fitzherbert, J. (1534) *The Boke of Husbandry*. London: Thomas Bethlet.

Fleming, G. (1871) *Animal Plagues: Their History, Nature and Prevention* (Volume One). London: Chapman & Hall.

——(1876) *The Contagious Diseases of Animals: Their Influence on the Wealth and Health of the Nation and How They are to be Combated*. London: Baillière, Tindall & Cox.

Fogle, B. (1981) *Interrelations between People and Pets*. Springfield: Charles C. Thomas.

Frey, E.F. (1985) 'The Earliest Medical Texts'. *Clio Medica*. 20: 1, pp.79–90.

Friedmann, E. (1995) 'The Role of Pets in Enhancing Human Well-being: Physiological Effects'. In Robinson, I. (ed.) *The Waltham Book of Human–Animal Interaction: Benefits and Responsibilities of Pet-Ownership*. Oxford: Pergamon. pp.33–54.

Friedmann, E., Katcher, A.H., Thomas, S.A., Lynch, J.J. and Messent, P. (1983) 'Interaction and Blood Pressure: Influence of Animal Companions'. *Journal of Nervous and Mental Disease*. 171, pp.461–5.

Gamgee, J. (1863) *The Diseases of Animals in Relation to Public Health and Prosperity: A Lecture*. Edinburgh: Maclachlan & Stewart.

——(1866) *The Cattle Plague; with Official Reports of the International Veterinary Congress held in Hamburg, 1863 and in Vienna 1865*. London: Robert Hardwicke.

Garnsey, P. (1988) *Famine and Food Supply in the Graeco-Roman World*. Cambridge: Cambridge University Press.

Gibson, W. (1738) *The Farrier's New Guide*.

Giddens, A. (1980) *Studies in Social and Political Theory*. London: Hutchinson.

Glickman, L.T. (1993) 'The Epidemiology of Human Toxocariasis'. In Lewis, J.W. and Maizels, R.M. (eds) *Toxocara and Toxocariasis: Clinical, Epidemiological and Molecular Perspectives*. London: Institute of Biology. pp. 3–10.

Gogolin-Ewens, K.J., Meeusen, E.N.T., Scott, P.C., Adams, T.E. and Brandon, M.R. (1990) 'Genetic Selection for Disease Resistance and Traits of Economic Importance in Animal Production'. *Revue Scientifique et Technique de l'Office International des Epizooties*. 9: 3, pp.865–96.

Goudsblom, J. (1986) 'Public Health and the Civilizing Process'. *Milbank Quarterly*. 64: 2, pp.160–88.

——(1989a) 'Human History and Long-Term Social Processes'. In Goudsblom, J., Jones, E.L. and Mennell, S. (eds) *Human History and Social Process*. Exeter: Exeter University Press. pp.11–26.

——(1989b) 'Ecological Regimes and the Rise of Organised Religion'. In Goudsblom, J., Jones, E.L. and Mennell, S. (eds) *Human History and Social Process*. Exeter: Exeter University Press. pp. 63–78.

——(1989c) 'The Formation of Military-Agrarian Regimes'. In Goudsblom, J., Jones, E.L. and Mennell, S. (eds) *Human History and Social Process*. Exeter: Exeter University Press. pp.79–92.

——(1990) 'The Impact of the Domestication of Fire upon the Balance of Power between Human Groups and other Animals'. *Focaal*. 13, pp.55–65.

——(1992) *Fire and Civilization*. Harmondsworth: Penguin.

Grimes, J.E. (1987) 'Zoonoses Acquired from Pet Birds'. *Zoonotic Diseases, Veterinary Clinics of North America: Small Animal Practice*. 17: 1, 209–18.

Hall, S.A. (1991) 'The State of the Art of Farriery'. *Veterinary History*.7: 1, pp.10–11.

Hammer, C.R. (1993) 'Medical Scientists must Vigorously Develop Xenografting as a Viable Clinical Alternative'. *Journal of Heart and Lung Transplantation*. 12: 6 (2), pp.360–4.

Harris, M. (1977) *Cannibals and Kings: The Origins of Culture*. New York: Vintage Books.

——(1985a) *Good to Eat: Riddles of Food and Culture*. New York: Simon & Schuster.

——(1985b) *Culture, People, Nature: An Introduction to General Anthropology* (Fourth Edition). New York: Harper & Row.

Harrison, R. (1964) *Animal Machines*. London: Stuart.

Hart, L.A. (1995) 'The Role of Pets in Enhancing Human Well-being: Effects for Older People'. In Robinson, I. (ed.) *The Waltham Book of Human–Animal Interaction: Benefits and Responsibilities of Pet-Ownership*. Oxford: Pergamon. pp.19–32.

Hayden, B. (1992) 'Contrasting Expectations in Theories of Domestication'. In Gebauer, A.B. and Price, T.D. (eds) *Transitions to Agriculture in Prehistory*. Madison, Wisconsin: Prehistory Press. pp. 11–19.

Hecker, H.M. (1982) 'Domestication Revisited: Its Implications for Faunal Analysis'. *Journal of Field Archaeology*. 9, pp.217–36.

Hemmer, H. (1990) *Domestication: The Decline of Environmental Appreciation*. [Translated by Beckhaus, N.: Original German Version Published 1983.] Cambridge: Cambridge University Press.

Hemsworth, P.H., Barnett, J.L. and Coleman, G.J. (1993) 'The Human–Animal Relationship in Agriculture and its Consequences for the Animal'. *Animal Welfare*. 2, pp.33–51.

Higgs, E.S. and Jarman, M.R. (1969) 'The Origins of Agriculture: A Reconsideration'. *Antiquity*. 43 (169), pp. 31–41.

Hobday, F.T.G. (1900) *Canine and Feline Surgery*. London: W. & A.K. Johnston.

Holst, P.A.J. (1991) *Bird Keeping as a Source of Lung Cancer and other Human Diseases: A Need for Higher Hygienic Standards*. Berlin: Springer-Verlag.

Hooper, W. D. and Ash, H.B. (Translators) (1934) *Cato and Varro: De Re Rustica*. London: William Heinemann.

Horzinek, M.C. and Zijpp, A.J. van der (1993) 'General Introduction to Biotechnology in Animal Breeding, Husbandry and Animal Health'. In Vuijk, D.H., Dekkers, J.J. and Plas, H.C. van der (eds) *Developing Agricultural Biotechnology in the Netherlands*. Wageningen: Pudoc. pp. 83–90.

Houwers, D.J. (1994) 'Brucella-DNA in een vroeg 15e-eeuwse Afvalput'. *Argos: Bulletin van het Veterinair Historisch Genootschap*. 11, p.27.

Hyams, E. (1972) *Animals in the Service of Man*. Philadelphia: J.B. Lippincott.

Hyland, A. (1990) *Equus: The Horse in the Roman World*. London: B.T. Batsford.

ID-DLO (1995) *Jaarverslag 1994*. Lelystad: ID-DLO.

Ingold, T. (ed.) (1988) *What is an Animal?* London: Unwin Hyman.

——(1994) 'From Trust to Domination: An Alternative History of Human–Animal Relations'. In Manning, A. and Serpell, J. (eds) *Animals and Human Society: Changing Perspectives*. London: Routledge. pp.1–35.

James, R. (1760) *A Treatise on Canine Madness*. London: J. Newbury.

Jarman, M.R. and Wilkinson, P.F. (1972) 'Criteria of Animal Domestication'. In Higgs, E.S. (ed.) *Papers in Economic Prehistory*. Cambridge: Cambridge University Press. pp. 83–89.

Johnson, A. (1991) *Factory Farming*. Oxford: Blackwell.

Jones, E.L. (1988) *Growth Recurring: Economic Change in World History*. Oxford: Clarendon Press.

Jones, J.M. (1992) *Food Safety*. St Paul, Minnesota: Eagan Press.

Kamp, M.D.O. van der (1994) *Ways of Replacing, Reducing or Refining the Use of Animals in the Quality Control of Veterinary Vaccines*. Lelystad: Institute for Animal Health and Science (ID-DLO).

Karasszon, D. (1988) *A Concise History of Veterinary Medicine*. (Trans. Farkas, E. and Kecskés, I.K.) Budapest: Akadémiai Kiadó.

Katcher, A.H. (1981) 'Interaction between People and their Pets: Form and Function'. In Fogle, B. (ed.) *Interrelations between People and Pets*. Springfield: Charles C. Thomas. pp.41–67.

Katcher, A.H. and Beck, A.M. (1983) *New Perspectives on Our Lives with Companion Animals*. Philadelphia: University of Philadelphia Press.

Kerstens, C.J.Q. (1971) 'How it Evolved'. In Willan, J.W. (ed.) *Veterinary Work in the Netherlands*. Leidschendam: Veterinary Service Information Division. pp.12–25.

Kete, K. (1994) *The Beast in the Boudoir: Pet-keeping in Nineteenth Century Paris*. Berkeley: University of California Press.

Koolmees, P.A. (1991) *Vleeskeuring en Openbare Slachthuizen in Nederland 1875–1985*. Utrecht: Stichting Histosearch.

——(1997) *Symbolen van Openbare Hygiëne: Gemeentelijke slachthuizen in Nederland 1795–1940*. Rotterdam: Erasmus.

Koolmees, P.A. and Mathijsen, A.H.H.M. (1993) 'The Development of Veterinary Medicine in the Netherlands: A Chronological Orientation'. *Argos: Bulletin van het Veterinair Historisch Genootschap*. 8, pp.233–47.

——(1996) 'Boekbespreking: Dunlop, R. and Williams, D. *Veterinary Medicine: An Illustrated History*'. *Argos*: *Bulletin van het Veterinair Historisch Genootschap*. 14, pp.159–61.

Kotula, A.W. (1991) 'By-Products'. In Putnam, P.A. (ed.) *Handbook of Animal Science*. San Diego: Academic Press.

Lacey, R. W. (1994) *Mad Cow Disease: History of BSE in Britain*. St Helier, Jersey: Cypsela.

Lane, J. (1993) 'Farriers in Georgian England'. In Michell, A.R. (ed.) *History of the Healing Professions: Parallels between Veterinary and Medical History* (Volume 3). London: C.A.B. International. pp.99–118.

Langdon, J. (1986) *Horses, Oxen and Technological Innovation: The Use of Draught Animals in English Farming from 1066 to 1500*. Cambridge: Cambridge University Press.

Lappin, M.R. (1993) 'Feline Zoonotic Diseases'. *Feline Infectious Diseases, Veterinary Clinics of North America: Small Animal Practice*. 23: 1, pp.57–78.

Lawrence, J. (1796) *A Philosophical and Practical Treatise on Horses and the Moral Duties of Man Towards the Brute Creation*. London: Longman.

Layard, D.P. (1762) *An Essay on the Bite of a Mad Dog*. London: Printed for John Rivington and Thomas Paynes.

Leach, E. (1964) 'Anthropological Aspects of Language: Animal Categories and Verbal Abuse'. In Lenneberg, E.H. (ed.) *New Directions in the Study of Language*. Cambridge, MA: MIT Press. pp. 23–63.

L'Estrange Ewen, C. (1933) *Witchcraft and Demonianism: A Concise Account Derived from Sworn Depositions and Confessions Obtained in the Courts of England and Wales*. London: Heath Cranton.

Levinson, B. (1972) *Pets and Human Development*. Springfield: Charles C. Thomas.

Lévi-Strauss, C. (1966) *The Savage Mind*. London: Weidenfeld & Nicolson.

Lewis, J.W. and Maizels, R.M. (1993) *Toxocara and Toxocariasis: Clinical, Epidemiological and Molecular Perspectives*. London: Institute of Biology.

Lloyd, S. (1993) '*Toxocara canis*: The Dog'. In Lewis, J.W. and Maizels, R.M. (eds) *Toxocara and Toxocariasis: Clinical, Epidemiological and Molecular Perspectives*. London: Institute of Biology. pp. 11–21.

Loar, M.G. (1987) 'Risks of Pet Ownership: The Family Practitioner's Viewpoint'. *Zoonotic Diseases, Veterinary Clinics of North America: Small Animal Practice*. 17: 1, 17–25.

Lobban, R.A. (1989) 'Cattle and the Rise of the Egyptian State'. *Anthrozoös*. 2: 3, pp.194–201.

——(1994) 'Pigs and their Prohibition'. *International Journal of Middle East Studies*. 26, pp.57–75.

Loew, F.M. (1990) 'Animals and People in Revolutionary France: Scientists, Cavalry, Farmers and Vétérinaires'. *Anthrozoös*. 4: 1, pp.7–13.

Macfarlane, A. (1970) *Witchcraft in Tudor and Stuart England: A Regional and Comparative Study*. London: Routledge & Kegan Paul.

McGlone, J.J., Nicholson, R.I., Hellman, J.M. and Herzog, D.N. (1993) 'The Development of Pain in Young Pigs Associated with Castration and Attempts to Prevent Castration-Induced Behavioral Changes'. *Journal of Animal Science*. 71, pp.1441–6.

McNeill, W.H. (1963 [1991]) *The Rise of the West: A History of the Human Community*. Chicago: University of Chicago Press.

——(1976) *Plagues and Peoples*. London: Penguin.

Maehle, A-H. (1994) 'Cruelty and Kindness to the "Brute Creation": Stability and Change in the Ethics of the Man–Animal Relationship, 1600–1850'. In Manning, A. and Serpell, J. (eds) *Animals and Human Society: Changing Perspectives*. London: Routledge. pp. 81–105.

Manchester, K. (1984) 'Tuberculosis and Leprosy in Antiquity: An Interpretation'. *Medical History*. 28, pp. 162–73.

Markham, G. (1648) *Cheape and Good Husbandry for the Well-ordering of all Beasts and Fowles and for the General Cure of their Diseases* (Seventh edition). London: Bernard Alsop.

Mason, J. and Singer, P. (1980) *Animal Factories*. New York: Crown.

Meadow, R.H. (1989) 'Osteological Evidence for the Process of Animal Domestication'. In Clutton-Brock, J. (ed.) *The Walking Larder: Patterns of Domestication, Pastoralism, and Predation*. London: Unwin Hyman. pp. 80–90.

Messent, P.R. and Serpell, J.A. (1981) 'An Historical and Biological View of the Pet-Owner Bond'. In Fogle, B. (ed.) *Interrelations between People and Pets*. Springfield: Charles C. Thomas. pp. 5–22.

Meyer, H. (1992) '10,000 Years "High on the Hog": Some Remarks on the Human–Animal Relationship'. *Anthrozoös*. 5: 3, pp.144–59.

Michaels, M.G. and Simmons, R.L. (1994) 'Xenotransplant-associated Zoonoses: Strategies for Prevention'. *Transplantation*. 57: 1, 1–7.

Midgley, M. (1983) *Animals and Why they Matter*. Athens: University of Georgia Press.

Ministerie van Landbouw, Natuurbeheer en Visserij (1992) *Intensieve Veehouderij*. Den Haag: Infotiek.

Ministry of Agriculture, Fisheries and Food (MAFF) (1965) *Animal Health: A Centenary 1865–1965*. London: HMSO.

Mol, J. (1971) 'The Organisation and Duties of the Regional Animal Health Services'. In Willan, J.W. (ed.) *Veterinary Work in the Netherlands*. Leidschendam: Veterinary Service Information Division. pp. 43–53.

Murray, J. (1830) *Remarks on the Disease called Hydrophobia*. London: Longman, Rees, Orme, Brown & Green.

Nutton, V. (1983) 'The Seeds of Disease: An Explanation of Contagion and Infection from the Greeks to the Renaissance'. *Medical History*. 27, pp.1–34.

Ockerman, H.W. and Hansen, C.L. (1988) *Animal By-product Processing*. Chichester: Ellis Horwood.

Offringa, C. (1971) *Van Gildenstein naar Uithof: 150 Jaar Diergeneeskundig Onderwijs in Utrecht. Deel I*. Utrecht: Faculteit der Diergeneeskunde.

——(1976) 'Van Empirist tot Dierenarts: de Creatie van een Beroep'. *Spiegel Historiael*. 11, pp.162–9.

——(1981) *Van Gildenstein naar Uithof: 150 Jaar Diergeneeskundig Onderwijs in Utrecht. Deel 2*. Utrecht: Faculteit der Diergeneeskunde.

——(1983) 'Ars Veterinaria: Ambacht, Professie, Beroep. Sociologische Theorie en Historische Praktijk'. *Tijdschrift voor Geschiedenis*. 96, pp.407–32.

Pattison, I. (1981) *John McFadyean*. London: J.A. Allen.

——(1984) *The British Veterinary Profession: 1791–1948*. London: J.A. Allen.

——(1990) *A Great British Veterinarian Forgotten: James Beart Simonds 1810–1904*. London: J.A. Allen.

Pharming (1995) *Pharming Health Care Products: Annual Report 1995*.

Porter, R. (1993) 'Man, Animals and Medicine at the Time of the Founding of the Royal Veterinary College'. In Michell, A.R. (ed.) *History of the Healing Professions: Parallels between Veterinary and Medical History* (Volume 3). London: C.A.B. International. pp.19–30.

Postgate, J. (1992) *Microbes and Man* (Third edition). Cambridge: Cambridge University Press.

Postma, O.H., Stranzinger, G., Strijker, R. and Went, D.F. (1996) 'Transgenic Dairy Mammals'. *Bulletin of the International Dairy Federation*. 315, pp.39–51.

Pugh, L.P. (1962) *From Farriery to Veterinary Medicine: 1785–1795*. Cambridge: W. Heffer & Sons.

Rackham, J. (1994) *Interpreting the Past: Animal Bones*. London: British Museum Press.

Redman, C.L. (1978) *The Rise of Civilization: From Early Farmers to Urban Society in the Ancient Near East*. San Francisco: W.H. Freeman.

Regan, T. (1983) *The Case for Animal Rights*. London: Routledge & Kegan Paul.

Reid, W. (1871) *Sheep: Their History, Management, Diseases and Nutritional Value, with Remarks of the Transit of Stock*. Edinburgh: William P. Nimmo.

Rifkin, J. (1992) *Beyond Beef: The Rise and Fall of the Cattle Culture*. New York: Dutton.

Rindos, D. (1984) *The Origins of Agriculture: An Evolutionary Perspective*. Orlando: Academic Press.

Ritvo, H. (1987a) *The Animal Estate: The English and other Creatures in the Victorian Age*. Cambridge, MA: Harvard University Press.

——(1987b) 'The Emergence of Modern Pet-Keeping'. *Anthrozoös*. 1: 3, pp.158–65.

Roberts, H.R. (1981) *Food Safety*. New York: John Wiley & Sons.

Robinson, I. (1995) *The Waltham Book of Human–Animal Interaction: Benefits and Responsibilities of Pet-Ownership*. Oxford: Pergamon.

Rutgers, L.J.E. (1993) *Het Wel en Wee der Dieren: Ethiek en Diergeneeskundig Handelen*. Doctoral Thesis: Rijksuniversiteit Utrecht.

Ryder, M.L. (1983) *Sheep and Man*. London: Duckworth.

Ryder, R. (1989) *Animal Revolution: Changing Attitudes towards Speciesism*. Oxford: Basil Blackwell.

Sagoff, M. (1996) 'Animals as Inventions: Biotechnology and Intellectual Property Rights'. *Institute for Philosophy and Public Policy*. 16: 1.

Sahlins, M. (1972) *Stone Age Economics*. London: Tavistock.

Sainsbury, D. (1986) *Farm Animal Welfare: Cattle, Pigs and Poultry*. London: Collins.

Salisbury, J.E. (1994) *The Beast Within: Animals in the Middle Ages*. New York: Routledge.

Schantz, P.M. (1990) 'Preventing Potential Health Hazards Incidental to the Use of Pets in Therapy'. *Anthrozoös*. 4: 1, pp.14–23.

Schenk, P. (1988) 'Het Dier als Voedsel: Van Extensieve naar Intensieve Veehouderij'. In Visser, M.B.H. and Grommers, F.J. (eds) *Dier of Ding: Objectivering van Dieren*. Wageningen: Pudoc.

Schwabe, C.W. (1978) *Cattle, Priest and Progress in Medicine*. Minneapolis: University of Minnesota Press.

——(1984a) *Veterinary Medicine and Human Health* (Third edition). Baltimore: Williams & Wilkins.

——(1984b) 'Drinking Cow's Milk: The Most Intense Man–Animal Bond'. In Anderson, R.K., Hart, B.L. and Hart, L.A. (eds) *The Pet Connection: Its Influence on Our Health and Quality of Life*. Minneapolis: University of Minnesota Press. pp.50–57.

——(1994) 'Animals in the Ancient World'. In Manning, A, and Serpell, J. (eds) *Animals and Human Society: Changing Perspectives*. London: Routledge. pp.36–58.

'Scottish Tenant Farmer' (1866) *On the Management of Farm Stock in Health and Disease*. Edinburgh: William Blackwood & Sons.

Serpell, J. A. (1987) 'Pet-keeping in Non-western Societies: Some Popular Misconceptions'. *Anthrozoös*. 1: 3, pp. 166–74.

——(1989) 'Pet-keeping and Animal Domestication: A Reappraisal'. In Clutton-Brock, J. (ed.) *The Walking Larder: Patterns of Domestication, Pastoralism, and Predation*. London: Unwin Hyman. pp.10–21.

——(1996) *In the Company of Animals: A Study of Human–Animal Relationships*. Cambridge: Cambridge University Press. (Revised edition: Original published 1986.)

Shadwell, J. (1790) 'Cases of Hydrophobia'. In Mease, J. (1793) *An Essay on the Disease produced by the Bite of a Mad Dog, or other Rabid Animal*. London: C. Dilly.

Sherratt, A. (1981) 'Plough and Pastoralism: Aspects of the Secondary Products Revolution'. In Hodder, I., Isaac, G. and Hammond, N. (eds) *Patterns of the Past: Studies in Honour of David Clarke*. Cambridge: Cambridge University Press. pp.261–305.

——(1983) 'The Secondary Exploitation of Animals in the Old World'. *World Archaeology*. 15: 1, pp.90–104.

Singer, P. (1990) *Animal Liberation: A New Ethics for Our Treatment of Animals*. New York: New York Review. (Revised edition: First published 1975.)

Singleton, W.B. (1993) 'Companion Animal Medicine: Future Outlook'. In Michell, A.R. (ed.) *Veterinary Medicine Beyond 2000*. Wallingford, Oxon: C.A.B. International. pp. 249–64.

Smith, F. (1919–33) *The Early History of Veterinary Literature and its British Development* (4 volumes; reprinted from *The Veterinary Journal*). London: J.A. Allen (Reprinted 1976).

——(1927) *A History of the Royal Veterinary Corps, 1796–1919*. London: Baillière.

Smith, H.S. (1969) 'Animal Domestication and Animal Cult in Dynastic Egypt'. In Ucko, P.J. and Dimbleby, G.W. (eds) *The Domestication and Exploitation of Plants and Animals*. London: Duckworth. pp. 307–14.

Smithcors, J.F. (1957) *Evolution of the Veterinary Art: A Narrative Account to 1850*. Kansas City: Veterinary Medicine Publishing.

Spackman, T. (1613) *A Declaration of such Grievous Accidents as Commonly Follow the Biting of Mad Dogges*. London: Printed for John Bill.

Spier, F. (1995) 'Norbert Elias' Theorie van Civilisatieprocessen Opnieuw ter Discussie: Een Verkening van de Opkomende Sociologie van Regimes'. *Amsterdams Sociologisch Tijdschrift*. 22: 2, pp.297–323.

——(1996) *The Structure of Big History: From the Big Bang until Today*. Amsterdam: Amsterdam University Press.

Steele, J.H. (1977) *Zoonoses as Occupational Diseases in Agriculture and Animal Related Industries*. Chicago: American Medical Association.

Stehr-Green, J.K. and Schantz, P.M. (1987) 'The Impact of Zoonotic Diseases Transmitted by Pets on Human Health and the Economy'. *Zoonotic Diseases, Veterinary Clinics of North America: Small Animal Practice*. 17: 1, 1–13.

Strickland Constable, H. (1866) *Observations Suggested by Cattle Plague about Witchcraft, Superstition and Parliamentary Reform and other Matters*. London: Dalton & Lucy.

Swaan, A. de (1985) *Het Medisch Regiem*. Amsterdam: Meulenhoff.

——(1988) *In Care of the State: Health Care, Education and Welfare in Europe and the USA in the Modern Era*. New York: Oxford University Press.

Swabe, J.M. (1994) 'Preserving the Emotional Order: The Display and Management of Emotion in Veterinary Interaction'. *Psychologie en Maatschappij*. 68: 3, pp.248–60.

——(1995) *Mad Dogs and Englishmen: A Tale of Humans, Hounds and Hydrophobia in Nineteenth Century Britain*. Unpublished paper presented at the British Sociological Association Conference, Leicester, UK, April 1995.

——(1996) 'Dieren als een Natuurlijke Hulpbron: Ambivalentie in de Relatie tussen Mens en Dier, binnen en buiten de Vétérinaire Praktijk'. In Heerikhuizen, B. van *et al.* (eds) *Milieu als Mensenwerk*. Groningen: Wolters-Noordhoff.

Sykes, M., Lee, L.A. and Sachs, D.H. (1994) 'Xenograph Tolerance'. In Möller, G. (ed.) *Immunological Reviews*. No. 141. Copenhagen: Munksgaard. pp.245–76.

Tabor, R. (1991) *Cats: The Rise of the Cat*. London: BBC Books.

Tambiah, S.J. (1969) 'Animals are Good to Think and Good to Prohibit'. *Ethnology*. 8, pp.424–59.

Tamminga, S., Spoelstra, S.F. and Kempen, G.J.M. van (1993) 'General Introduction to Biotechnology in Animal Nutrition'. In Vuijk, D.H., Dekkers, J.J. and Plas, H.C. van der (eds) *Developing Agricultural Biotechnology in the Netherlands*. Wageningen: Pudoc. pp.169–74.

Tannenbaum, J. (1989) *Veterinary Ethics*. Baltimore: Williams & Wilkins.

Tester, K. (1991) *Animals and Society: The Humanity of Animal Rights*. London: Routledge.

Thomas, K. (1983) *Man and the Natural World: Changing Attitudes in England 1500–1800*. London: Penguin.

Topsell, E. (1607) *The Historie of Foure-Footed Beastes*.

Toynbee, J.M.C. (1973) *Animals in Roman Life and Art*. London: Thames & Hudson.

Trümpler, U., Straub, P.W. and Rosenmund, A. (1989) 'Antibacterial Prophylaxis with Lactoferrin in Neutropenic Patients'. *European Journal of Clinical Microbiological Infectious Disease*. 8, pp.310–13.

Tuan, Y. (1984) *Dominance and Affection: The Making of Pets*. New Haven: Yale University Press.

Tudge, C. (1993) *The Engineer in the Garden: Genetics: From the Idea of Heredity to the Creation of Life*. London: Pimlico.

Ucko, P.J. and Dimbleby, G.W. (1969) 'Introduction: Context and Development of Studies of Domestication'. In Ucko, P.J. and Dimbleby, G.W. (eds) *The Domestication and Exploitation of Plants and Animals*. London: Duckworth. pp. xvii–xxi.

Underman, A.E. (1987) 'Bite Wounds Inflicted by Dogs and Cats'. *Zoonotic Diseases, Veterinary Clinics of North America: Small Animal Practice*. 17: 1, pp.195–207.

Veenman, F.M.C. (1995–1997) *Veterinairrechtelijke Voorschriften EG (Gezondsheids en Welzijnswet voor Dieren)*. Lelystad: Koninklijke Vermande.

Visser, H.K.A. (1996) 'Human Lactoferrine'. *Tijdschrift voor Jeugdgezondheidszorg*. 28: 3, pp.40–44.

Visser, I.J.R. (1996) 'De Georganiseerde Dierziektenbestrijding in de 18e, 19e en begin 20e Eeuw in Nederland'. *Argos: Bulletin van het Veterinair Historisch Genootschap*. 14, pp.135–52.

Visser, M.B.H. and Grommers, F.J. (eds) (1988) *Dier of Ding: Objectivering van Dieren*. Wageningen: Pudoc.

Voith, V. (1981) 'Attachment between People and their Pets: Behavioural Problems that Arise from the Relationship between Pets and People'. In Fogle, B. (ed.) *Interrelations between People and Pets*. Springfield: Charles C. Thomas.

Vries, J. de (1984) *European Urbanization 1500–1800*. London: Methuen.

Waal, D. de (1987) *Welzijn van Dieren in Nederland*. 's Gravenhage: Staatsuitgeverij.

Walker, R.E. (1973) 'Roman Veterinary Medicine'. In Toynbee, J.M.C. *Animals in Roman Life and Art*. London: Thames & Hudson.

Ward, K.A., Nancarrow, C.D., Byrne, C.R., Shanahan, C.M., Murray, J.D., Leish, Z., Townrow, C., Rigby, N.W., Wilson, B.W. and Hunt, C.L.H. (1990) 'The Potential of Transgenic Animals for Improved Agricultural Productivity'. *Revue Scientifique et Technique de l'Office International des Epizooties*. 9: 3, pp.847–64.

Webster, J. (1994) *Animal Welfare: A Cool Eye Towards Eden*. Oxford: Blackwell.

Weijden, G.C. van der and Rozendal, A. (1995) 'Historische Aspecten van de Verloskunde van het Rund'. *Argos: Bulletin van het Veterinair Historisch Genootschap*. 13, pp.81–6.

West, G.P. (ed.) (1961) *A History of the Overseas Veterinary Services*. London: British Veterinary Association.

Wester, J. (1939) *Geschiedenis der Veeartsenijkunde*. Utrecht: Hoonte.

White, R. (1862) *Doubts about Hydrophobia as a Specific Disease to be Communicated by the Bite of a Dog*. London: Knight & Lacey.

White, R.G., DeShazer, J.A., Tressler, C.J., Borcher, G.M., Davey, S., Waninge, A., Parkhurst, A.M., Milaunk, M.J. and Clemens, E.T. (1995) 'Vocalisation and Physiological Response of Pigs During Castration With or Without a Local Anesthetic'. *Journal of Animal Science*. 73, pp. 381–6.

Wilkinson, L. (1984) 'Rinderpest and Mainstream Infectious Disease Concepts in the Eighteenth Century'. *Medical History*. 28, pp.129–50.

——(1992) *Animals and Disease: An Introduction to the History of Comparative Medicine*. Cambridge: Cambridge University Press.

——(1994) 'Craft to Science: Animal Diseases in Veterinary Science'. In Arnold, K. (ed.) *Animal Doctor: Birds and Beasts in Medical History*. Exhibition catalogue: Wellcome Institute for the History of Medicine.

Willis, R. (ed.) (1990) *Signifying Animals: Human Meaning in the Natural World*. London: Routledge.

Wilmut, I., Schnieke, A.E., McWhir, J., Kind, A.J. and Campbell, K.H.S. (1997) 'Viable Offspring Derived from Fetal and Adult Mammalian Cells'. *Nature*. 385, pp.810–13.

Winkler, J.K. (1982) *Farm Animal Health and Disease Control*. Philadelphia: Lea & Febiger.

Winnicott, D.W. (1980) *Playing and Reality*. Harmondsworth: Penguin.

Wiseman, J. (1986) *A History of the British Pig*. London: Duckworth.

Wood, J. (1814) *General Conclusions of the Nature and Cure of Hydrophobia, Intended for Popular Reading*. Newcastle: E. Walker.

Worboys, M. (1992) 'Killing and Curing: Veterinarians, Medicine and Germs in Britain, 1860–1900'. *Veterinary History*. 7: 2, pp.53–71.

Wray, C. and Woodward, M.J. (1990) 'Biotechnology and Veterinary Science: The Production of Veterinary Medicines'. *Revue Scientifique et Technique de l'Office International des Epizooties*. 9: 3, pp.779–94.

Youatt, W. (1830) *On Canine Madness*. London: Longman.

——(1845) *The Dog*. London: Charles Knight & Co.

Zeuner, F.E. (1963) *A History of Domesticated Animals*. London: Hutchinson.

Zivanovic, S. (1982) *Ancient Diseases: The Elements of Palaeopathology*. [Translated by Edwards, L.F.] London: Methuen.

INDEX

Ackerknecht, E.H. 109
Adamson, P.B. 63–4, 213–14
affective dependency 18, 191
agrarianisation 17, 23–4, 46, 70, 85
agrarian regime 23, 39–40
agrarian society 39–44, 62–70, 73, 85, 113, 169
agribusiness 118, 122, 124
agriculture 17, 24–31, 39–41, 44–5, 52–5, 57, 59, 66, 68, 70, 74, 85–6, 89–91, 101, 105, 118–21, 124, 147, 194; Common Agricultural Policy 147–8; origins of 17, 24–31;
Agricultural Society of Odiham 91
Albertus Magnus 81, 169, 172
anaesthetics 130–2, 152, 179
ancient societies: Egypt 53–5, 62–5, 71–2, 213; Greek society 55–6, 65, 72–3, 75, 162; Mesopotamia 50, 52–3, 62–3, 70–1; Roman society 55–7, 65–6, 72–6, 169, 171
Anderson, B.K. 185
Anderson, J.K. 56
Anderson, R.M. 215
animal by-products 2–4, 34, 51–2 140, 206–12
animal disease control: 97–105, 108, 129, 138–9, 141–2, 148–51, 184, 187–8, 195, 202, 205; British legislation 98, 100–1, 114, 143, 150; Dutch legislation 101–3, 116, 143, 145; globalisation of 150–1; harmonisation of measures 148–9; international 106, 142, 148–51; state intervention; 17, 98–104, 107–8, 114–15, 142–51; *see also* vaccination
animal domestication 10, 13, 16–17, 23–39, 42, 46–7, 175, 201; impact on human social life 10, 23, 38–44; theories on 28–38
animal feed 54, 63, 119–22, 127, 133, 137, 140–1, 192, 206–11, 214; animal feed industry 121, 153; animal nutrition 95, 123, 131, 133, 152, 155, 170, 190, 202
animal husbandry 10, 16, 23, 39–41, 45, 50, 52, 68–9, 85–6, 120, 128, 146, 157, 201–3; artificial insemination 146; embryo transfer 134, 195; in vitro fertilisation 195; management of animal reproduction 15, 155, 182, 195
animal medicine *see* veterinary medicine
animal plagues *see* epizootics
animal rights 7, 9, 87, 134, 193
animal skins *see* hide
animal sanctuaries 180, 184
animal symbolism 6–7, 54, 163
animals: in ancient societies 53–7, 162, 171; attitudes towards 7–10, 57, 101, 163; for

companionship 5, 160–1, 168; disposal of dead 2–3, 69, 96–7, 100, 103, 114; in the early modern period 57, 59–62, 163–6; for entertainment and sport 5, 56, 58, 72, 161; experimentation on 4–5, 161, 168–9, 196, 198; exploitation of 7–10, 17–18, 42, 44, 49–52, 57–60, 70, 86, 117, 125, 137, 192–4, 203–5; human dependency on 1–7, 11, 18, 23, 30, 40–2, 49, 52–3, 62, 70, 85, 137, 155, 191–3; increasing sensibilities to 163–4, 178, 193; in the Middle Ages 57–60, 162, 166, 170, 172; as a natural resource 7, 9–10, 18, 30,193, 204; in the New World 60; patenting of 196; as pharmaceutical factories 197; philosophical thought 7–9, 58, 89; role of in human society 1–7, 156, 192–4, 204; as status symbols 167; theological view of 7–9, 58; use for traction 9, 24, 34, 50–1, 55–6, 58, 67, 81, 92, 114, 180; transportation of: 95, 120, 140–2, 147–9; *see also* individual species
animal waste 122, 135–8, 185–8; *see also* dung, manure, pet animal excreta
animal welfare 2, 9, 14, 17, 124–37, 145, 147–8, 157, 168, 184, 192–3, 200, 201, 203
antelopes 35–6
anthrax 49, 52, 57, 64–6, 68–9, 90, 104, 109–14, 140, 144, 150, 215; vaccine 111–12, 144
anthropomorphism 53, 158, 160
antibiotics 123, 127, 131, 137–9, 152; use as growth promoters 129, 138–9, 192
acquired immune deficiency syndrome (AIDS) 187, 193, 198
Armelagos, G.J. 29
Ash, E.C. 166, 171, 174
Ash, H.B. 57, 74–5
asses 50, 56
aurochs 21, 35
automobiles 151–2, 190
Australia 59, 61, 106, 120, 199
Azzaroli, A. 55–6

Baarda, B. 185
bacon 129
bacteriology 94, 109–12, 143–5
Baker, J. 19–20
Baker, S. 6
Bakewell. R. 61
Ballarini, G. 90
Barclay, H.B. 56
Barker, G. 28, 57
Barnard, C. 197
Bates, T. 84
battery egg production 118, 125–8
Beattie, C.P. 187
Beck, A.M. 185
beef 60–1, 106, 120, 132–4, 148, 181; tinned beef 106
Bentham, J. 9
Bertin, H-L. 90
Bieleman, J. 84, 121
birds 72, 100, 170; avian zoonoses 189–9; falconry 170; as pets 5, 35, 178–9, 188–9, 191; wild 1, 139, 189
biopharmaceuticals 18, 196–7, 199–200, 203–4
biotechnology 18, 123, 193, 195, 200, 202, 204–5
Bisseru, B. 186
blacksmiths 77, 80, 94, 178
Blaine, D.P. 174–7
Blaisdell, J.D. 64
Blake, N.F. 81
Blancou, J. 80–1, 194–5
Blood, D.C. 141
Bodson, L. 72–3, 76
Bøkønyi, S. 32, 36, 38
Bonner, J. 139
Boor-van der Putten, I.M.E. 169–70, 174–5, 177–9
Boserup, E. 28
Bourdieu, P. 7
Bourgelat, C. 90
Bouw, J. 165

bovine pleuropneumonia 69, 87, 96–7, 102, 104, 114, 143
bovine somatotropin (BST) 133, 195–6
bovine spongiform encephalopathy (BSE) 4, 133, 146–7, 149–50, 193, 205, 207, 214–5
Bowler, J. 3
Bracken, H. 79
Brander, G.C. 138–9
Brauell, F. 110
Brock, T.D. 83, 110–12
Broom, D.M. 130
Brothwell, D. 19–20, 49, 51, 62
brucellosis (contagious abortion) 62, 140, 145–6, 155, 215; vaccine 145
Budiansky, S. 30, 37–40
Burden, W. 78
Burnet, M. 22, 44
Byzantine Empire 76

Caius, J. 162–3, 166, 174
Callis, J. 202
calves 59, 72, 123, 131–4, 140, 146, 181, 201, 214; *see also* cattle, veal
Cantley, M.F. 200
Cavalieri, P. 198
camels 34, 50, 213; camelids 213
Campbell, K.H.S. 199
campylobacteriosis 139–40
canine distemper 48, 173–5, 183
castration: of cattle 56; of dogs 170; of pigs; castrators 131, 170, 214
cats 5, 35, 38, 156, 158–9, 161, 165, 165, 175–6, 178–9, 181, 183, 186–8, 190–1, 203; breeding of 165; castration of 175–6; cat litter 187–8; cat scratch fever 188; feline disease 175, 186–8; feline medicine 181; feline panleukopenia 175, 181, 183; for vermin control 158, 168
Cato the Elder 74
cattle 1, 20–1, 30–1, 34–5, 37, 47–8, 50–1, 53–6, 58–61, 63, 68–9, 72, 75, 82, 84–5, 96–7, 100, 102, 106, 118–19, 124, 131–4, 136, 140–1, 146, 156, 179, 195–6, 203; Belgian Blue 134, 202; cattle wealth 53–4; cloning of 199–200; dehorning of 132–4, 155, 203; transgenesis in 196–7, 203
cattle culture 12, 53–5, 72
cattle plague 17, 82–4, 88–9, 94, 99, 104–7, 117, 147; in Britain 17, 88, 96, 99–101, 107; in the Netherlands 17, 88–9, 101–4; *see also* rinderpest
Charnock Bradley, O. 12
Chaucer, G. 81
chemotherapy 182
chickens 1, 35, 60, 111, 118, 124–6, 202–3; battery hens 118, 125, 127–8; broiler chickens 126–127, 129, 139, 202; debeaking 127, 132, 134, 203; *see also* eggs, poultry
Childe V. G. 27–8, 39
chlamydia infections 141, 189; ornithosis 189; psittacosis 189
Christianity 7–9, 57–8, 89; crusades 77; monastic orders 81
classical swine fever 131, 145, 149–50, 193, 215
Clater, J. 174
Clayton, B. 172
cloning 18, 199–200; Dolly the Sheep 199; Megan & Morag 199; Roslin Institute 199
Clutton-Brock, J. 21, 26–7, 30–5, 38, 55, 76
Cockburn, A. 46
Cohen, M. N. 28–9
Coleman, E. 92–3, 176
Columella, L.J.M. 75, 169, 171
consumer food demands 60, 62, 86, 96, 105, 119–21, 126, 132, 135, 141, 156, 193, 195, 202
contagious disease *see* infectious disease
contagionism *see* germ theory
Cothchin, E. 12
cow-leeches 82, 88, 94, 107

cowpox 48, 111; cowpox vaccine 111
Crosby, A.W. 60
CSS report 5, 158, 185
Cunningham, W. 113

Daems, W. 200
dairying 51, 57, 85, 140
dairy produce 1, 49, 51, 56, 60, 121, 132, 140, 144, 147; *see also* milk
D'Arcy Thompson, R. 12
Davids, K. 60, 120, 123–4, 180
Davis, S.J.M. 25, 30, 35–6, 51–2, 60, 157
Dekkers, M. 6
Delafond, H.M.O. 110
Descartes, R. 8
Diamond, J. 52
Dimbleby, G.W. 26, 28, 38
Dixon, K.R. 55
disease transmission 19–23, 45–9, 65, 74–5, 92, 104–5, 126, 136–8, 140–2, 176, 186–9, 214; contagion 75, 83–4, 92, 95, 142, 173; spontaneous generation 83, 97, 109, 172–3, 176
dogs 5–6, 33–5, 37, 48–50, 56–7, 72, 100–1, 112, 134, 156–9, 161, 163–6, 168–79, 181, 183, 185–6, 188, 190–1, 203; breeding of 164–7; bites from 171–3, 188; castration of 170; diseases of 72, 112, 167, 169–74, 76, 183, 186; lap-dogs 159, 161–4, 166; licenses for 167; tail-docking 171, 177, 216; working dogs 6, 50, 56–7, 161, 164, 166, 168
Dolan, T.M. 167
domestication *see* animal domestication, fire domestication, plant domestication
donkeys 5, 34–5, 50, 56
dormice 57
Douglas, M. 6
Doyen-Higuet, A-M. 76
Driesch, A. von den 212
Dubey, J.P. 187
dung 51–2, 169, 213; medicinal uses of 52, 169
Dunlop, R. 11, 56, 61, 67, 76–7, 81–4, 89, 110, 112, 115, 145, 152, 171, 178–9, 181

early modern period 57, 59–62, 68–70, 77–87
E.Coli 136, 193
eggs 1, 3, 19, 85, 121–2, 125, 212; *see also* battery egg production
El-Ahraf, A.L. 135, 137
Elias, N. 14–15, 41, 87, 164
Ellis, P.R. 138–9
empirics 72–3, 88–9, 94, 102
Endenburg, N. 159–60, 185
Enlightenment, the 88, 165
environment 2, 17, 124, 135–137, 151, 184, 187–8, 192, 196; environmental nuisance 185–7; nitrate pollution 137
epidemics 17, 45, 47, 65–8, 104, 106; *see also*plague
epizootics 17, 52, 65–70, 81, 83–4, 87–91, 95–106, 147–8, 150, 214
equestrianism 42–3, 55, 77, 81
equine medicine 72, 75–80, 90, 93, 151–2, 174, 181
ethnography 15, 29
European Union (EU) 130, 133, 139, 147–9, 159, 196; European parliament 130
euthanasia 182, 184
extensive farming practice 119–20, 122–3; extensification 148
extensive growth 28, 70

factory farming *see* intensive farming practice, livestock production
farcy *see* glanders
farriery 77–80, 88, 91–2, 94, 107
Ferrando, R. 90
ferrets 35
Fiddes, N. 1, 7, 21

Fiennes, R. N. T-W. 20, 45, 48, 189
fire, domestication of 13, 26, 44, 85
fish 2, 5, 72, 212
Fischer, K-D. 76, 212
Fischer-Homberger, E. 109
Fisher, J.R. 4, 12, 88–94, 98, 101, 107–8
Fitzherbert, J. 69
Flanders 59
fleas 169, 184
Fleming, G. 65, 67, 96, 214
Fogle, B. 185
Food and Agricultural Organisation 150
food-borne infection 19–21, 45, 63–4, 113, 115, 138–40, 193, 216
food chain 22, 138, 155
food safety 116, 138, 140–1, 148–9
foot-and-mouth disease 69, 83, 87, 96–7, 104, 144–5; vaccine 144
fowl cholera 110–11; vaccine 111
foxes 5, 134
Fracastoro, G. 83
France 58, 61, 67, 90–1, 93, 101, 105, 132, 147, 166; French Revolution 115
Frank, J.P. 114–15
Frederick II 77
free-range farming 134–5
Frenkel, H.S. 144
Frey, E.F. 71
Friedmann, E. 185

Galen 75, 83
Galton, F. 33
Gamgee, J. 96–100, 104
Garnsey, P. 65
Gaultier, P-V. 111–12
gelatine 2–4, 110, 208
gelders 94,178
genetics: DNA 62, 196, 199, 202; eugenics 164; genetic engineering 194–5, 200–1, 203, 205; genetic manipulation 18, 165–6, 202–3; gene mapping 194; molecular genetics 193–4; pleiotropy 201; recombinant DNA technology 194–5, 202–3; *see also* transgenesis
germ theory 75, 97, 99, 102, 109, 112
Gibson, W. 79
glanders 80–1, 90, 92–3, 104, 114, 214
Glickman, L.T. 186
goats 30, 34–5, 51–2, 56–7, 74, 119, 124, 156, 196; use of hair 52
Gogolin-Ewens, K.J. 195
Goudsblom, J. 13, 25–6, 30, 39–40, 42–3, 85, 87, 214
Great Britain 16, 59–61, 80, 83–4, 86, 89, 91, 93, 95, 97, 100, 102, 104–7, 113, 117, 120, 126, 131–2, 143, 147, 166, 176–7, 179, 215; Central Veterinary Laboratory 145–7; Ministry of Agriculture, Fisheries and Food (MAFF) 96–9, 101, 105–6, 114, 146–7; Royal College of Veterinary Surgeons 107–8, 176; State Veterinary Service 145–7
Grisone, F. 77
Grimes, J.E. 189
Guinea-pigs 35, 182, 188

habitus 7, 143, 183, 215
Hall, S.A. 78
Hammer, C.R. 198
Hansen, C. L. 2–4
Harris, M. 6, 24, 31, 64, 212
Harrison, R. 131
Hart, L.A. 185
Hayden, B. 29
Hecker, H. M. 32, 36
Hemmer, H. 38
Hemsworth, P.H. 135
Hengeveld, G.J. 102
hide 2–3, 7, 19–20, 31, 44, 51, 59–60, 97, 102, 150, 206, 208, 210, 213
Higgs, E.S. 31
Hobday, F. 179–80

Holst, P.A.J. 189
Homer 65
hominids 19, 24, 26, 44
Hooper, W.D. 57, 74–5
Hope, W. 79
hormone use 4, 138, 149
horse marshals 77
horses 1, 5–6, 34–5, 37, 43, 47, 51, 58, 60, 69, 78, 90, 92–3, 151–2, 156, 168, 174, 177–80; agricultural usage 58–60; hippotherapy 5; horseshoeing 76, 90; military use of 6, 55, 58, 60, 75–7, 79–80, 92–3, 151, 174, 213; *see also* equestrianism, equine medicine
Horzinek, M.C. 194–5
Houwers, D.J. 62
human-animal relationships 7–10, 12–14, 16–18, 22–3, 25–6, 31–2, 38, 44–6, 57–8, 63, 85–8, 137, 151, 156–8, 160, 163, 168, 184–5, 190–4, 204, 212; ambiguous nature of 157, 161; human-animal interdependence 12, 14–15, 22,105
humans; socio-cultural development of 24–28, 38–9
humoral pathology 73–4, 112, 175
hunter-gatherers 24–5, 27, 29–30, 39–41, 157; marginalisation of 39, 41, 50
hunting 5, 19, 21, 23–27, 31–3, 43–44, 56, 58, 72, 161, 170; game drives 21, 27, 34; hunting dogs 6, 161–4,166, 170
hyaena 34
Hyams, E. 34
Hyland, A. 55

immunology 112, 123, 143, 152
industrialisation 17, 85–7, 117, 120, 163; of agricultural production 91
infectious disease 10, 17, 40, 57, 62, 68, 80, 83, 85, 89, 96–7, 100, 102, 104, 109, 123, 125–6, 131, 134, 137–8, 140, 143, 152–3, 171, 183, 185, 189, 193, 198; emergence of 44–9; *see also*disease transmission, epidemics, epizootics, plague, zoonotic disease
influenza 48, 67
Ingold, T. 6
insects 5, 212
insulin 4, 178, 198
intensive growth 70
intensive farming practice 118–42, 146, 148–9, 156, 192–3, 203
internal combustion engine 151, 180, 190
international veterinary cooperation 98, 105, 147–151; Office International des Epizooties 147
Italy 67, 69, 81, 83, 132, 147, 187

Jakob, H. 179
James, R. 173
Jarman, M. R. 31–2
Jenner, E. 111
Johnson, A. 9, 118–20, 122–3, 125–6, 130, 132–3, 136–8, 140, 149, 216
Johnson, K.G. 130
Jones, J.M. 70, 139, 143
Judaism 53, 63; Jews 99

Kahun papyrus 71
Kamp, M. D. O. van der 5
Karasszon, D. 11, 72–4
Katcher, A.H. 185
Kerstens, C.J.Q. 90, 102–3, 143
Kete, K. 166
Kircher, A. 83
knackers 114, 151
Koch, R. 109–10
Koolmees, P.A. 11–12, 21, 87, 114–16, 144, 150
Kotula, A.W. 4, 206–11
Kòchenmeister, F. 115

Lacey, R.W. 4
lamb 120
lambs 57, 123
Lancisi, G.M. 84

land enclosure 86, 119
Lane, J. 80
Langdon, J. 58, 60
Lappin, M.R. 186–7
Lawrence, J. 78–80
Layard, D.P.
lay-healers 81–2, 95; *see also* empirics
Leach, E. 7
leather 141
Leeuwenhoek, A. van 83, 109
leptospirosis 136, 140–1, 183
L'Estrange Ewen, C. 69
Leuckart, R. 115
Levinson, B. 185
Lévi-Strauss, C. 6
Lister, J. 112
listeriosis 140
livestock 9–10, 30–1, 41–3, 65–9; breeding 51, 61, 120, 127, 134, 195; housing of 119, 121–8, 132, 134–6, 138, 141, 155; importation of 69, 95–9, 102, 105, 120, 142, 148; livestock-keeping 30, 33, 51, 60, 157, 215; transportation of 95, 142
livestock husbandry *see* animal husbandry
livestock production 89, 98, 119, 121, 195; intensification of 17, 60, 118–42
Livy 66
Lloyd, S. 186
Loar, M.G. 191
Lobban, R.A. 54, 63–4
Loew, F.M. 90

Macfarlane, A. 69
McNeill, W.H. 14, 42, 44–9, 54–5, 62–3, 65–8, 213
Maehle, A-H. 8–9
Manchester, K. 20, 48, 63
mange 175
Manure 4, 59, 100, 121; poultry manure 140; *see also* dung
Markham, G. 79, 82
Marshall plan 144
Mason, J. 126–8, 131, 139
mastitis 133, 136, 155
Matthijsen, A.H.H.M. 12
Mayhew, E. 179
Meadow, R. H. 23, 32
measles 48, 174
meat 1–2, 19–20, 20–1, 30–1, 33, 39, 49 51, 56, 59–61, 63, 97, 102, 106, 115, 120–2, 126, 129–30, 134, 140, 144, 149, 154, 186, 192, 200, 213–4; boar taint 129–30; meat hygiene 20–1, 114; meat inspection 12, 113–16, 130, 144, 149, 152, 180, 214
mediaeval Europe 57–60, 66–8, 75–7, 81–2, 162, 166, 170, 172, 213
Messent, P.R. 158
Meyer, H. 64
Michaels, M.G. 198–9
microparasites 22, 25
Midgley, M. 7
milk 2–3, 34, 39–40, 49, 51–2, 57, 59–60, 85, 109, 119, 122–3, 132–3, 140, 144, 195–6, 200–1, 203; asses milk 56; lactoferrin 196–7, 200; pasteurisation of 110, 155
Mol, J. 144
molecular biology 62
monopolisation of violence 14, 43, 87
mules 56
mulomedici 76
Murray, J. 173

Neoteny 37, 159
Netherlands, the 11, 15, 60, 86, 89, 96, 101–2, 104, 107, 114, 116–17, 119–20, 123, 126, 130–2, 136, 143, 149, 179, 187, 196, 215; Animal Health Services 144; Austrian Netherlands 84; Centraal Bureau voor Statistiek 124; Central Veterinary Institute 145; domestic animal population of 124; Dutch sociology 11, 13; farm waste crisis 136–7; Friesland 144;

Ministerie van Landbouw, Natuurbeheer en Visserij 130,145; Rijksveeartsenijschool 95, 102, 108, 144, 179; State Serum Institute 143–145; State Veterinary Research Institute 144–5
Newcastle disease 190, 193
New Zealand 59, 61, 106, 120
North America 106, 177 *see also* United States
Numan, A. 94
Nutton, V. 75, 83

Ockerman, H. W. 2–4
Offringa, C. 12, 89–91, 94–5, 102–3, 107–9, 112, 115, 144–5, 178, 180, 190
oryx 34
oxen 50, 56, 58, 75, 99

palaeopathology 50, 62
parasites 20–1, 23, 42, 45–7, 52, 62, 68, 73, 115, 169, 175, 183, 189, 191; *see also* microparasites
parasitology 115, 143, 145, 152
parvo virus 183
pastoralism 41–2, 53
Pasteur, L. 109–12, 173
pasturellosis
Pattison, I. 12, 79, 88, 91, 93
personality structure 14, 87, 164
pets 5–6, 18, 33, 35, 57, 124, 152, 154, 156–91, 198, 202, 214; allergies to 188–9; breeding of 159, 164–6, 195, 202; cute response to 159; exotic pets 35; neutering of 155, 184; pet animal excreta 78, 185–8, 191; pet food 180, 187, 190, 216; pet industry 168, 180, 184–5; pets and human health 184–91; pet psychology 190; pet therapy 185; as transitional objects 158–9
pet-keeping 18, 33, 35, 152, 156–68, 174, 177, 180, 184, 188, 191, 202; explanations for 157–60; history of 160–8
Petri, R. 110
Phebus, G. 170
pigs 1, 20, 30, 35, 56–7, 60–1, 63–4, 72, 85, 115, 118–19, 123–4, 130, 133, 149, 156, 196, 198–9, 203; castration of 57, 129–31, 136, 138; intensive pig farming 128–31, 138, 149, 215; organs for transplantation 198–9; tail-docking 118, 129, 132, 134
plague 73, 83, 189; of Athens 65; Black Death 67–8; *see also* epidemic disease, epizootics
plants, domestication of 25–8, 31, 45
Pliny, the elder 171–2
Poels, J. 143
pork 61, 63–4, 120, 129; food taboo 63–4
Porter, R. 91, 94, 178
Postgate, J. 22
Postma, O.H. 196
poultry 85, 119, 123–8, 131, 133, 138–9, 145, 156, 189–90, 214; *see also* chickens, turkeys
poultry production 123–8, 139–40
power relations 25, 29, 39, 43
predation 19, 21–3, 27, 44, 134–5
primates 26, 198, 214
process sociology 11, 13–14
proto-professionalisation 183
psittacosis
public health 18, 104, 113–14, 116, 124, 136, 138–9, 145, 148–9, 152, 157, 168, 173, 184–5, 191–2, 202, 205, 214–5; public health management 153
Pugh, L.P. 11, 77–8, 82, 88

quarantine 68, 74–5, 84, 100, 173, 190

rabies 49, 66, 101, 104, 111–12, 167–8, 171–3, 183, 188, 190; post-exposure vaccine 112, 173
rabbits 35, 112, 182, 188, 191
Rackham, J. 24

Ramazzini, B. 84
Redman, C.L. 28
refrigeration 1, 106, 142
Regan, T. 7–9
Reid, W. 60
regimes, concept of 9–10
religion 8, 21, 24, 42, 53–4, 71–2, 161, 212; bible 7–8, 59, 64; role of priests 42–3, 71, 214; *see also* Christianity, Judaism
reptiles 5, 35, 182, 189
Rifkin, J. 60
rinderpest 48, 66–7, 69, 83–4, 87, 89, 96, 99–106, 114–15; losses from 101, 103–4, 174; *see also*cattle plague
Rindos, D. 30, 36–7
ringworm 141
Ritvo, H. 101, 164–7, 173
Robinson, I. 185
rodents 182, 188–9
Rozendal, A. 72
Ruffus, J. 77, 80
Rutgers, L.J.E. 134
Ryder, M.L. 56–7, 61
Ryder, R. 125

Sagoff, M. 196
Sainsbury, D. 125, 127–8, 134, 136, 138
St. Bel, C.V. de 91–3, 174, 176, 214
St. Hildegard 81
Salisbury, J.E. 58–9, 213
salmonella 136, 139–40, 155, 189, 193
scabies 104, 170
scrapie 145, 215
Schantz, P.M. 188–9
schistosomiasis 62–4
Schenk, P. 119, 122
Schwabe, C.W. 12, 48, 51, 53–4, 71–2, 76, 113, 140–1, 186–7, 213
secondary animal produce 10, 51–2; *see also* milk, dung, hide
sedentism 27–8, 44–5
selective breeding 60–1, 190, 201, 214
Serpell, J. A. 8, 33, 158–9, 161–3, 190
sheep 1, 30, 34–5, 37, 47, 52–3, 56–7, 59–61, 63, 67, 72, 96, 99, 111–12, 119, 124, 133, 156, 187, 196, 213; cloning of 199; diseases of 66–7, 90, 97, 104, 111, 187; sheep-pox 90, 97, 104; Spanish Merino 61; *see also*lamb, wool
Sherratt, A. 50–1
silage 132–3, 137
Simmons, R.L. 198–9
Simonds, J.B. 93, 106
Singer, P. 4, 7, 118, 124, 126–8, 130–3, 139, 198, 215
Singleton, W.B. 183
slaughterhouses 3, 12, 87, 96, 114–15, 130, 140, 154, 215; slaughterhouse by-products 2–4, 206–11; waste 139
slurry 118, 136–7
smallpox 48, 67, 84, 89, 111
Smith, F. 11–12
Smith, H.S. 35
Smithcors, J.F. 11, 73, 75
social organisation 10, 26–7, 41, 47
social relations 10, 16–17, 23, 27, 32–3, 38–44, 53–5, 87, 160; competition 29, 42; cooperation 27, 32–3; interdependence 14–15, 41; self control 10, 14, 41, 87; social control 14, 41 87; social differentiation 14, 29, 39, 42, 54, 166–7; social stratification 39, 166
Solleysel, J.L. de 77, 79–80
Southern, P. 55
Spackman, T. 172–3
Spain 58, 61, 147
specific pathogen free (SPF) animals 139, 145, 199
Spier, F. 11
state formation 87; in ancient Egypt 54, 63–4
state, role of: 17, 88, 91, 97–9, 107–8, 114–17
state veterinary services 143;

Britain 99, 107, 145–7; Netherlands 104, 108, 116, 143–5
Stehr-Green, J.K. 189
Steel, J.H. 177
Steele, J.H. 48, 66, 140–1, 151, 189
stockmen 135, 141
Strickland Constable, H. 99–100
Swaan A. de 104, 183
Swabe, J.M. 7, 15, 101, 167, 173, 182, 190
Sykes, M. 198

tail-docking 118, 129, 132, 134, 155, 171, 177, 216
Tambiah, S. J. 6
Tamminga, S. 195
Tannenbaum, J. 129–30, 133
tapeworms 20, 114–15
Tester, K. 7
Thomas, K. 8, 59, 61, 85, 123, 162–4, 213
Topsell, E. 81
tongue-worm 171–2
Toussaint, J-J. H. 111
toxacariasis 186, 188
toxoplasmosis 20, 140, 181, 186–8
Toynbee, J.M.C. 56
transgenesis: 194, 196–7, 199–200, 203–4
transgenic animals 194, 196–7, 199–200, 203; Herman the bull 196–7; 'oncomouse' 196
trichinosis 64, 114–15, 140, 215
Trümpler, U. 197
Tuan, Y-F. 157
tuberculosis (including bovine variant) 20, 48–9, 62–3, 111, 114, 116, 140, 144–5, 150, 155, 181, 215
Tudge, C. 194, 201, 203
tularemia 20
turkeys 35, 60, 126, 202

Ucko, P.J. 26, 28, 38
Underman, A.E. 188
United Kingdom *see* Great Britain
United States 123–4, 126, 131, 133, 149, 198
urbanisation 17, 54, 86, 113, 120–1, 159, 163

vaccines 4, 111, 123, 144–5, 149, 152, 173, 181, 195, 202, 204
vaccination 99, 111, 123, 125, 138, 141, 146, 173, 183, 184, 191
variolation 89
Varro 74–5
veal 57, 123, 131–2
Veenman, F.M.C. 149
vegetarianism 1, 3; veganism 212
Vegetus Renatus 76
vellum 3, 59
veterinarians 15, 92, 101–3, 106–8, 110, 116, 131–2, 140–4, 146, 148, 151–5, 177–9, 182–3, 191, 204; army 92–3, 104, 180–1; inspectors: 104, 108, 113, 146, 148–9; large animal practitioners 151–5; para-veterinarians 131, 214; popular image of 183; relationship with farmers; 94, 102, 106–7, 112, 116, 142, 148, 154; small animal practitioners 152, 154, 168, 182–4, 191
veterinary drug residues 138, 155
veterinary education 17, 89–95, 107–8, 112, 152–3, 179; Britain 91–4; Denmark 90; France 90; Germany 91, 108–9; London Veterinary College 91–3, 106, 174, 176–7, 179–80, 214; Rijksveeartsenijschool 95, 102, 108, 144, 179; veterinary schools and colleges 12, 89–95, 107, 152–3, 178
veterinary history 11–12, 77, 175, 212
veterinary medicine 11, 18, 49, 97, 112–13, 174, 180, 194, 204; early animal medicine 70–84; equine medicine 72, 75–80, 90,

93, 151–2, 174, 181; laboratory animal science 153; large animal medicine 124, 151–5, 181; obstetrics 71–2, 134, 153, 155; small animal medicine 152, 156, 168–77, 179–84, 191; specialisation 157; wild animal medicine 153
veterinary profession 12, 17, 70, 88–9, 94–5, 100, 107–9, 112, 116–17, 151–2, 154, 168, 178, 181, 191; legislation pertaining to 107–8, 145, 148; social emancipation of 116–17
veterinary public health 113–17, 147, 149, 152–3, 157
veterinary regime 10–12, 13, 16–18, 49, 52, 104, 109, 118, 142–51, 155–6, 168–84, 190–1, 204–5; extension of to small animals 168–84, 190–1; formalisation of 17, 88, 116; globalisation of 150–1; informal veterinary regime 70–84; institutionalisation of 117; intensification of 17, 49, 85–118, 142–51, 157, 184; phaseology of 13
Villemin, J-A. 116
Virchow, R. 115
Virgil 65–6
Visser, H.K.A. 197
Visser, I.J.R. 104
Voith, V. 159
Vries, J. de 86

Waal, D. de 124–6, 130–1
Walker, R.E. 57, 76
Ward, K.A. 196
Webster, J. 119, 122, 124, 126–7, 133–4, 139
Weil's disease *see* leptospirosis
Weijden, G.C. van der 72
West, G.P. 12
Wester, J. 11
White, D.O. 22, 44
White, R. 173
White, R.G. 130
Williams, D. 11, 56, 61, 67, 76–7, 81–4, 89, 110, 112, 115, 145, 152, 171, 178–9, 181
Willis, R. 6
Willis, W.V. 135, 137
Wilkinson, P. F. 31–2
Wilkinson, L. 12, 49, 64, 67–9, 74, 81, 83–4, 93, 109, 111–12, 176, 214
Winkler, J.K. 215
Wiseman, J. 62
witchcraft 68–9, 99, 161; necromancy 165
wolves 27, 33–5, 48, 157, 165
Wood, J. 173
Woodward, M.J. 195, 202
wool 3–4, 51–2, 56–7, 59–61, 112–13, 213; cashmere 52
Worboys, M. 96, 100, 214
World Health Organisation 150
Wray, C. 195, 202

xenotransplantation 18, 197–9, 203–4
x-ray technology 152, 179

Youatt, W. 166, 173, 176–7

Zenker, F.A. 115
zero-grazing 132
Zeuner, F.E. 31
Zijpp, A.J van der 194–5
Zivanovic, S. 46–8, 62
zoocentrism 53
zoonotic disease 48–9, 64, 67, 80, 110, 112–13, 115–16, 140, 168, 198, 202